Atlas of Osteoarthritis

Nigel Arden, Francisco J. Blanco, Cyrus Cooper, Ali Guermazi,
Daichi Hayashi, David Hunter, M. Kassim Javaid, Francois Rannou,
Jean-Yves Reginster, Frank W. Roemer

This book has been published in partnership with the European Society for Clinical and Economic Aspects of Osteoporosis, Osteoarthritis and Musculoskeletal Diseases (ESCEO).

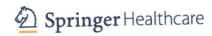

SWIMS

C20344606

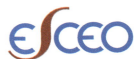

Published by Springer Healthcare Ltd, 236 Gray's Inn Road, London, WC1X 8HB, UK.

www.springerhealthcare.com

© 2014 Springer Healthcare, a part of Springer Science+Business Media.

British Library Cataloguing-in-Publication Data.
ISBN 978-1-910315-15-6 (Print)   978-1-910315-16-3 (eBook)

A catalogue record for this book is available from the British Library.

This publication has been made possible through an educational grant from SERVIER.

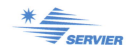

Atlas of Osteoarthritis

Nigel Arden

Musculoskeletal Epidemiology Unit & Oxford
Musculoskeletal BioBank
Oxford Biomedical Research Unit
University of Oxford, UK

Francisco J. Blanco

INIBIC-Hospital Universitario A Coruña
Universidad de Santiago de Compostela, Spain

Cyrus Cooper

Medical Research Council Lifecourse
Epidemiology Unit
University of Southampton, UK
National Institute for Health Research,
Musculoskeletal Biomedical Research Unit
University of Oxford, UK

Ali Guermazi

Quantitative Imaging Center
Boston University School of Medicine, USA

Daichi Hayashi

Quantitative Imaging Center
Boston University School of Medicine, USA

David Hunter

University of Sydney; Royal North Shore Hospital
North Sydney Orthopaedic and Sports Medicine
Centre, Australia

M. Kassim Javaid

University of Oxford, UK

Francois Rannou

Paris Descartes University; Cochin Hospital
Institut National de la Santé et de la Recherche
Médicale, France

Jean-Yves Reginster

Center for Investigation in Bone and Articular
Cartilage Metabolism
University of Liège, Belgium

Frank W. Roemer

Quantitative Imaging Center
Boston University School of Medicine, USA
Department of Radiology
University of Erlangen-Nuremberg, Germany

Contents

Contents

Author biographies

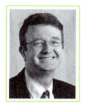

Nigel Arden, MBBS, FRCP, MSc, MD, is Professor of Rheumatology, Director of the Musculoskeletal Epidemiology Unit and the Oxford Musculoskeletal BioBank, he is also Deputy Director of the Oxford Biomedical Research Unit at Oxford University.

Professor Arden trained at St Thomas's Hospital, London, where he also completed four years of research into the genetics of osteoporosis. During this time, he gained an MSc in Epidemiology and an MD. In 1998 he spent six months as Visiting Professor in Epidemiology at the University of San Francisco.

In February 2000 he commenced his post as Consultant Rheumatologist at Southampton General Hospital, and Senior Lecturer in Rheumatology at the University of Southampton. He became a Professor of Rheumatic Diseases in Southampton in 2008 and at the University of Oxford in 2011. He is a Member of the National Osteoporosis Society Scientific Advisory Board; he is an International Osteoporosis Foundation Scientific Ambassador and sits on the European League Against Rheumatism (EULAR) Osteoarthritis Guideline Committee and the Osteoarthritis Research Society International (OARSI) Guidelines Committee. He has published over 200 research papers and 5 books.

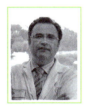

Francisco J. Blanco, MD, PhD, is Director of Research in the Biomedical Research Center of A Coruña (INIBIC) and Associate Professor of Medicine at the Universidad de Santiago de Compostela, Galicia, Spain. He was a Research Fellow at the University of California San Diego, USA.

Currently, Dr Blanco works as a rheumatologist in clinic at the Hospital Universitario A Coruña. His research group is focused on the cellular and molecular mechanisms of osteoarthritis, and on the search of biomarkers useful for diagnosis, prognosis and therapeutic response of rheumatic diseases. He is President of the Research and Training Committee of OARSI. He is a member of the CIBER-BBN (Bioengineer, Biomaterials and Nanomedicine) and the Proteo-Red (Spanish Network of Proteomics). Dr Blanco is Director of the Catedra-Bioiberica at A Coruña University and a member of the Editorial Board of the *Osteoarthritis and Cartilage, Arthritis Research and Therapy, Open Arthritis Journal, Open Proteomics Journal* and *Reumatologia Clínica*.

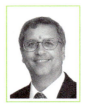

Cyrus Cooper MA, DM, FRCP, FFPH, FMedSci, is Professor of Rheumatology and Director of the Medical Research Council (MRC) Lifecourse Epidemiology Unit; Vice-Dean of the Faculty of Medicine at the University of Southampton; and Professor of Musculoskeletal Science at the University of Oxford.

Professor Cooper leads an internationally competitive programme of research into the epidemiology of musculoskeletal disorders, most notably osteoporosis. His key research contributions have been: discovery of the developmental influences which contribute to the risk of osteoporosis and hip fracture in late adulthood; demonstration that maternal vitamin D insufficiency is associated with sub-optimal bone mineral accrual in childhood; characterisation of the definition and incidence rates of vertebral fractures; and leadership of large pragmatic randomised controlled trials of calcium and vitamin D supplementation in the elderly as immediate preventative strategies against hip fracture. He is Chairman of the Committee of Scientific Advisors, International Osteoporosis Foundation; Chair of the MRC Population Health Sciences Research Network; Associate Director of Research at the University of Southampton Medical School; and Associate Editor of *Osteoporosis International*. He has published extensively (over 550 research papers) on osteoporosis and rheumatic disorders and pioneered clinical studies on the developmental origins of peak bone mass.

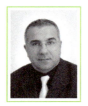

Ali Guermazi, MD, PhD, is a radiologist with expertise in imaging of musculoskeletal diseases. Currently, he is Professor of Radiology, Section Chief of Musculoskeletal Imaging and Director of the Quantitative Imaging Center at Boston University School of Medicine. He leads a research group focusing on the application of magnetic resonance imaging (MRI) to epidemiological studies and musculoskeletal radiology. He has been involved in developing several original and widely-accepted radiological methods to assess osteoarthritis disease risk and progression. He has also contributed to a number of large-scale multicentre osteoarthritis trials, such as the Multicentre Osteoarthritis Study, Health ABC, Framingham Osteoarthritis Study and Osteoarthritis Initiative.

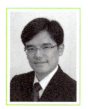

Daichi Hayashi, MBBS, PhD, is a radiologist-in-training and is currently a Research Assistant Professor of Radiology at Boston University School of Medicine. He completed his medical degree at King's College London School of Medicine, UK, and obtained his doctoral degree from Jikei University School of Medicine, Tokyo, Japan. He has been involved in musculoskeletal research, focusing on osteoarthritis and cartilage imaging for several National Institutes of Health (NIH) and pharmaceutical sponsored studies. His research interest includes MRI of musculoskeletal diseases, with a focus on osteoarthritis.

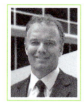

David Hunter, MBBS, PhD, FRACP, is Professor of Medicine at University of Sydney and Staff Specialist Rheumatologist at Royal North Shore Hospital and North Sydney Orthopaedic and Sports Medicine Centre. He completed his medical degree at the University of New South Wales (UNSW), a fellowship in Rheumatology at the Royal Australian College of Physicians, earned a Masters of Medical Science (Clinical Epidemiology) from the University of Newcastle, a Masters of Sports Medicine from UNSW and a PhD from the University of Sydney.

In his current work, Dr Hunter is investigating a number of key elements in osteoarthritis including the epidemiology of osteoarthritis, genetic epidemiology of osteoarthritis, the role of biomarkers in understanding osteoarthritis aetiopathogenesis, the application of imaging to better understand structure and function with application to both epidemiologic research and clinical trials, the application of novel therapies in disease management and heath service system delivery of chronic disease management. He is currently a board member of OARSI. Dr Hunter has over 200 peer reviewed papers published in international journals, numerous book chapters, has co-authored a number of books, including two books on self-management strategies for the lay public.

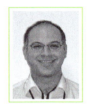

M. Kassim Javaid, MBBS, BMedSci, MRCP, PhD, Senior Research Fellow in Metabolic Bone Disease; Honorary Consultant and Rheumatologist at the University of Oxford. Dr Javaid completed his medical training at Charing Cross and Westminster Medical School and specialised in adult rheumatology at the Wessex Deanery. During that time, he also completed a PhD examining the maternal determinants of intra-uterine bone growth as part of an Arthritis Research Campaign (ARC) Clinical Fellowship at the University of Southampton. He was awarded an ARC travelling fellowship and worked with the osteoarthritis group in University of California San Francisco to study the role of vitamin D and bone in lower limb osteoarthritis.

Dr Javaid further extended his research into the role of vitamin D status in musculoskeletal disease, improving outcomes after fragility fracture as well as continuing work looking into the bone phenotypes in osteoarthritis. Balancing clinical and teaching, his direction of research is evermore linking the basic science with the key clinical issues in osteoarthritis and osteoporosis.

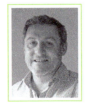

Francois Rannou MD, PhD, is Professor of Medicine at Paris Descartes University and Cochin Hospital. He is qualified in rehabilitation and rheumatology. He leads an INSERM (Institut National de la Santé et de la Recherche Médicale) team working in the field of cartilage and intervertebral disc biology. His clinical activity is mainly focussed on osteoarthritis and low back pain from care to randomised controlled trials.

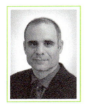

Frank W. Roemer, MD, is Co-Director of the Quantitative Imaging Center of the Department of Radiology at Boston University and Section Chief of MRI at the Department of Radiology at Klinikum Augsburg, a major teaching hospital in southern Germany. He holds academic appointments as Associate Professor at Boston University and the University of Erlangen, Germany, and is Associate Editor of *Osteoarthritis Cartilage* and *BMC Musculoskeletal Disorders.*

Dr Roemer is a German board-certified musculoskeletal radiologist with a strong focus on MRI. His main research interest is imaging of degenerative joint disease, sports imaging and imaging applications in pre-clinical research.

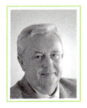

Jean-Yves Reginster, MD, PhD, is Professor and Chairman of Public Health Sciences, Epidemiology, and Health Economics at the University of Liège, where he also heads the Center for Investigation in Bone and Articular Cartilage Metabolism.

Professor Reginster trained at the University of Liège in Belgium, and specialised in physical medicine and rehabilitation (Liège), in public health (Nancy, France) and in epidemiology (Ann Arbor, MI, USA). He is President of the European Society for Clinical and Economic Aspects of Osteoporosis and Osteoarthritis, and of the Group for the Respect of Ethics and Excellence in Science. He is the General Secretary of the Belgian Bone Club. He is the co-founder of the International Osteoporosis Foundation where he currently serves on the Executive Committee, Board of Directors, Committee of Scientific Advisors and as Chairman of the Committee of National Sciences. Professor Reginster serves on the Editorial Boards of numerous journals, such as *Osteoporosis International, Bone* and *Calcified Tissue International*. He has written more than 600 scientific articles in the most distinguished journals (*New England Journal of Medicine, Lancet, Journal of Clinical Investigation, Journal of Endocrinology and Metabolism*) and more than 80 books or book chapters.

He is particularly interested in metabolic bone diseases, in the epidemiology, prevention, and treatment of postmenopausal osteoporosis and osteoarthritis, in all aspects of pharmacoepidemiology, public health and health economics, quality of life and in the methodology of clinical trials.

Chapter 1
Introduction: historical and current perspectives on osteoarthritis

Jean-Yves Reginster

Osteoarthritis is an important issue for both the individual and society [1], and its public health impact continues to grow due to the ageing population, the rising prevalence of obesity and the lack of definitive treatments to prevent or halt the progress of the disease [2]. However, osteoarthritis is difficult to define, and a better understanding of its pathophysiology is required [1,2].

What all forms of osteoarthritis and related disorders have in common is a loss of cartilage associated with bone features such as osteophytes and subchondral bone sclerosis [3]. However, the history of osteoarthritis is controversial because of its similarity to conditions such as diffuse idiopathic skeletal hyperostosis and ankylosing spondylitis as well as confusion between generalised osteoarthritis and osteoarthritis secondary to single traumatised joints. The terminology has been changing as well; over the years, osteoarthritis has been known as osteoarthrosis, degenerative joint disease, arthrosis deformans and morbus (malum) coxae senilis, among other terms [3].

Despite these difficulties, the occurrence of the disease across history is perhaps one of the best documented because of the persistence of bones compared with other bodily tissues [3,4]. The earliest examples of osteoarthritis in any animal are preserved in the bones of two dinosaurs approximately 100 million years old; microscopic examination has revealed increased vascular spaces and overgrowth of the articular margins [3]. The pathological characteristics of osteoarthritis have consequently remained unchanged [3], and it could be argued that the disease is an immutable part of life [5].

History of osteoarthritis in the literature

From the time of **Hippocrates** until approximately 250 years ago, all forms of chronic arthritis were considered to be manifestations of gout (Figure 1.1) [3,6]. The first break with that understanding came in 1782, when **William Heberden** described the nodes that now bear his name, highlighting that "they have no connexion with gout" [7].

One of the earliest physicians to describe a non-inflammatory erosion of the articular cartilage particular to the elderly was **Benjamin Brodie** in 1829 [8]. A further leap in understanding came with the description of osteoarthritis of the hip by **Robert Smith** in 1835 [9]. However, debate over the nature of the disease continued even after the coining of the term 'osteoarthritis' by **AE Garrod** in 1890 [3].

This publication has been made possible through an educational grant from SERVIER.

N. Arden et al., *Atlas of Osteoarthritis*, DOI 10.1007/978-1-910315-16-3_1,
© Springer Healthcare 2014

The introduction of X-rays at the end of the 19th century further enhanced our understanding of the disease process [3], while the linking of Heberden noduli with osteoarthritis by **Kellgren and Moore** in 1952 allowed the differentiation between generalised osteoarthritis and secondary osteoarthritis of a single traumatised joint [10]. The radiographic scoring system developed by **Kellgren and Lawrence** later that decade paved the way for them and others to provide a descriptive epidemiology of the condition [11,12].

Understanding of cartilage in the literature

Crucial to the developing knowledge of the processes of osteoarthritis was an understanding of the nature and function of articular cartilage. The first recorded description of articular cartilage

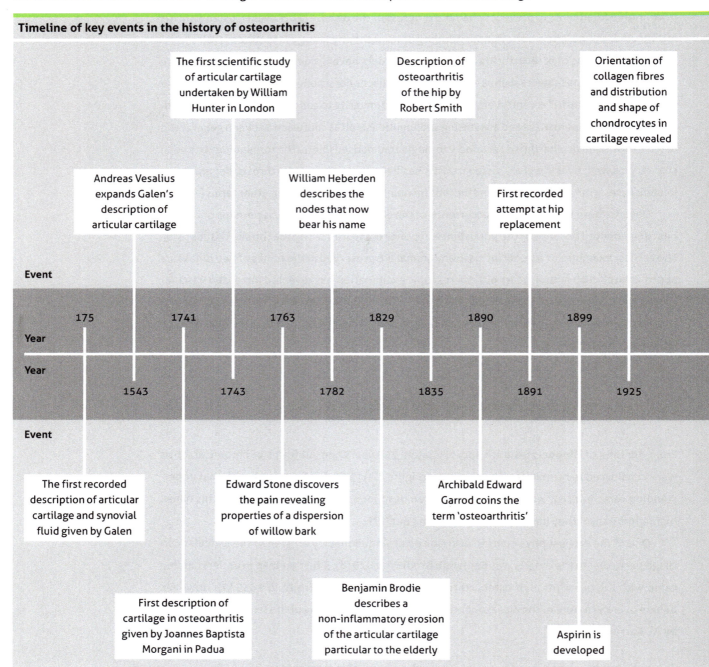

Timeline of key events in the history of osteoarthritis

The first scientific study of articular cartilage undertaken by William Hunter in London

Description of osteoarthritis of the hip by Robert Smith

Orientation of collagen fibres and distribution and shape of chondrocytes in cartilage revealed

Andreas Vesalius expands Galen's description of articular cartilage

William Heberden describes the nodes that now bear his name

First recorded attempt at hip replacement

Event

Year					
175	1741	1763	1829	1890	1899

Year

Year

1543	1743	1782	1835	1891	1925

Event

The first recorded description of articular cartilage and synovial fluid given by Galen

Edward Stone discovers the pain revealing properties of a dispersion of willow bark

Archibald Edward Garrod coins the term 'osteoarthritis'

First description of cartilage in osteoarthritis given by Joannes Baptista Morgani in Padua

Benjamin Brodie describes a non-inflammatory erosion of the articular cartilage particular to the elderly

Aspirin is developed

was given by **Galen** in his treatise from 175 AD titled *On the Usefulness of Various Parts of the Body* [13]. Alongside a discussion of synovial fluid, he describes cartilage thus [14]:

> " *Cartilages are spread on some parts of them [bones], such as the joints, to make them smooth, and Nature also uses cartilages occasionally as moderately yielding bodies... Cartilage serves as a grease for the joints.* "

Galen

In the 16th century, **Andreas Vesalius** substantially added to Galen's definitions, stating that cartilage "has no sensation and no marrow", but his crucial observation was that cartilage changes with age, such that it hardens and resembles "the fragility and friability of bone" [13].

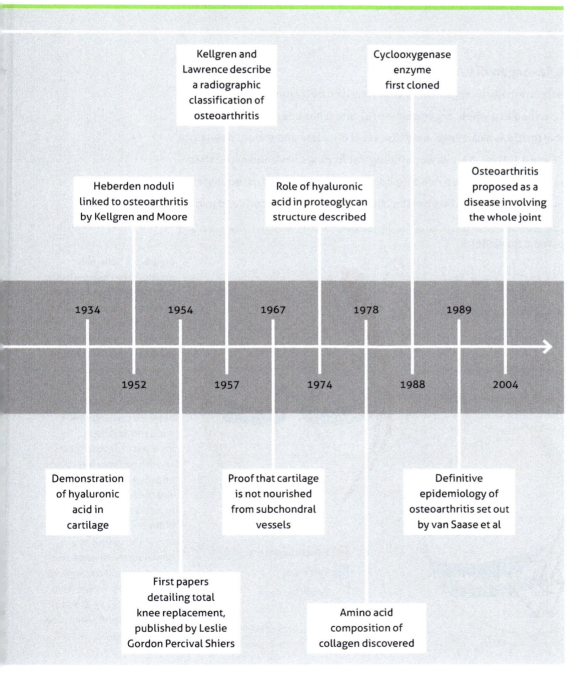

Figure 1.1 Timeline of key events in the history of osteoarthritis. Data from Dequeker & Luyten [3] and Benedek [6].

Kellgren and Lawrence describe a radiographic classification of osteoarthritis

Cyclooxygenase enzyme first cloned

Heberden noduli linked to osteoarthritis by Kellgren and Moore

Role of hyaluronic acid in proteoglycan structure described

Osteoarthritis proposed as a disease involving the whole joint

1934　1954　1967　1978　1989

1952　1957　1974　1988　2004

Demonstration of hyaluronic acid in cartilage

Proof that cartilage is not nourished from subchondral vessels

Definitive epidemiology of osteoarthritis set out by van Saase et al

First papers detailing total knee replacement, published by Leslie Gordon Percival Shiers

Amino acid composition of collagen discovered

The first description of cartilage in osteoarthritis was given by Joannes Baptista Morgagni in Padua in 1741, which was swiftly followed by what is considered to be the first scientific study of articular cartilage by William Hunter in London in 1743 [13]. Hunter's description opened up the debate as to how an apparently nerveless tissue lacking in blood supply could be nourished and grow. It was only with the development of enzyme chemistry that the pathophysiology of cartilage deterioration could be properly explored [13].

The first half of the 20th century saw two major discoveries: that cartilage could be divided into three layers through the orientation of collagen fibres and the distribution and shape of chondrocytes and that hyaluronic acid was found in cartilage. It is only in the last 30 years that our sophisticated understanding of collagen could be elucidated, through the use of immunological and enzyme analyses [13].

Osteoarthritis as a whole-organ disease

Although osteoarthritis has traditionally been primarily characterised by hyaline cartilage loss, it has more recently been described as a whole organ disease [3], and it has been suggested that the traditional view of osteoarthritis as a cartilage-only disease is obsolete and should open up to include the entire joint (Figure 1.2) [15,16]. Paleopathological findings have indicated that bony involvement in osteoarthritis may involve not only bone sclerosis, but also osteophytes and enthesophytes, which are ossifications of the insertion sites of ligaments, tendons and joint

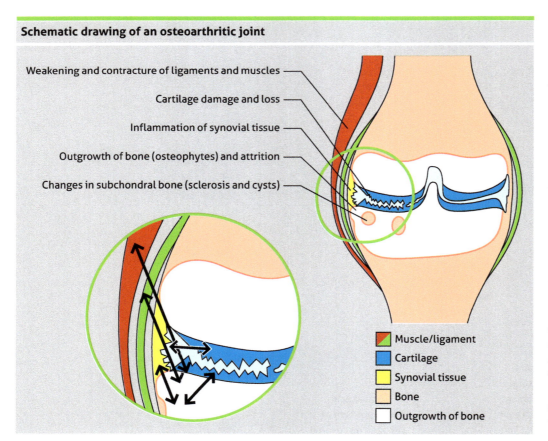

Schematic drawing of an osteoarthritic joint

Weakening and contracture of ligaments and muscles

Cartilage damage and loss

Inflammation of synovial tissue

Outgrowth of bone (osteophytes) and attrition

Changes in subchondral bone (sclerosis and cysts)

■ Muscle/ligament
■ Cartilage
■ Synovial tissue
■ Bone
□ Outgrowth of bone

Figure 1.2 Schematic drawing of an osteoarthritic joint. The different tissues involved in clinical and structural changes of the disease are shown on the left. Note that cartilage is the only tissue not innervated. On the right the bidirectional interplay between cartilage, bone and synovial tissue involved in osteoarthritis and the two-way interaction between this interplay and the ligaments and muscles are shown. In the bidirectional interplay, one of the tissues might dominate the disease and as such should be targeted for treatment. Image from Bijlsma et al [15]. © 2011, reproduced with permission from Elsevier.

capsule to the bone [17,18]. It is therefore likely that common molecular pathways regulate bone formation in different cellular niches, with osteophytes and enthesophytes potentially triggered by local joint stresses and abnormal mechanical joint loading [3].

Results from several studies have supported the whole-organ view of osteoarthritis. For example, synovitis is considered a pivotal factor in the pathogenesis of osteoarthritis, as suggested by the clinical symptoms of inflammation, the presence of histological inflammation in synovial tissue and early cartilage lesions at the border of the inflamed synovium [16]. There is also a correlation between degeneration of the anterior cruciate ligament and cartilage, particularly in the medial compartment of the knee joint [19]. Bone marrow lesions, commonly resulting from traumatic knee injuries, are significantly associated with pain in people with knee osteoarthritis [20].

Furthermore, there is growing evidence that subchondral bone plays an important role in osteoarthritis, with bone remodelling occurring preferentially in the subchondral plate, particularly in early-stage osteoarthritis [21]. This potentially makes the subchondral plate less able to absorb and dissipate energy [2]. These changes, alongside increases in bone volume [21], lead to increases in forces transmitted throughout the joint [2]. The structural progression of osteoarthritis may also be viewed primarily as an atheromatous vascular disease of subchondral bone [1].

The changing epidemiology of osteoarthritis

Historical comparisons have indicated that while the prevalence of osteoarthritis has increased substantially over the last few centuries, the clinical patterns have not. Waldron compared the prevalence of osteoarthritis in Georgian and early Victorian London with that of today, conducting an analysis of the skeletons of 360 men and 346 women, which were recovered from a church crypt used for burials between 1729 and 1869 [21]. Osteoarthritis of the large joints was comparatively uncommon, with osteoarthritis of the hip found in 1.1% of men and 2.9% of women and osteoarthritis of the knee in 0.8% of men and 5.2% of women [22]. Bilateral knee osteoarthritis was much more common in women than in men. The right side was affected in five of nine women and both men with unilateral disease (Figure 1.3, see page 14) [22].

The same author conducted a study of 115 cases and controls, matched for age and sex, of skeletons with osteoarthritis of the hands that were buried in London in the late 18th and early 19th centuries. Cases and controls were assessed for the presence of knee osteoarthritis. The skeletons with osteoarthritis of the hands had an almost sixfold increased likelihood of knee osteoarthritis versus controls, a significant odds ratio [23]. This pattern confirms the association observed in contemporary populations [23–25].

Our assumptions about the changing epidemiology of osteoarthritis may also be affected by discoveries about the pathophysiology of the disease that have led to a potential division of

Percentage distribution of different sites affected by knee osteoarthritis, by side affected

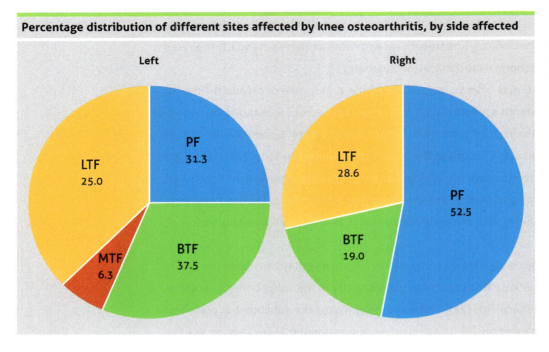

Figure 1.3 Percentage distribution of different sites affected by knee osteoarthritis, by side affected. On the left side, the disease was more or less equally likely to affect only patellofemoral compartment, only the lateral compartment, or both tibiofemoral compartments together. On the right side, the patellofemoral compartment was affected in slightly more than half the cases. The medial tibiofemoral compartment was affected alone in one case only. BTF, Both tibiofemoral compartments; LTF, lateral tibiofemoral compartment; MTF, medial tibiofemoral compartment; PF, patellofemoral compartment. Image from Waldron [22]. © 1991, reproduced with permission from the British Medical Journal Publishing Group.

the disease into distinct phenotypes (Table 1.1) [15]. In addition to improving our understanding of the disease, classifying the different clinical and structural phenotypes of osteoarthritis will allow for more direct targeting of treatments, depending on whether the predominate structural changes are in cartilage, bone, or synovial tissue. Nevertheless, there is currently no consensus on the subgrouping of osteoarthritis into these phenotypes, and they are not yet fully characterised [15].

Differentiation of clinical osteoarthritis phenotypes

	Post-traumatic (acute or repetitive)	Metabolic	Ageing	Genetic	Pain
Age	Young (<45 years)	Middle-aged (45–65 years)	Old (>65 years)	Variable	Variable
Main causative feature	Mechanical stress	Mechanical stress, adipokines, hyperglycaemia, oestrogen/progesterone imbalance	AGE, chondrocyte senescence	Gene related	Inflammation, bony changes, aberrant pain perception
Main site	Knee, thumb, ankle, shoulder	Knee, hand, generalised	Hip, knee, hand	Hand, hip, spine	Hip, knee, hand
Intervention	Joint protection, joint stabilisation, prevention of falls, surgical interventions	Weight loss, glycaemia control, lipid control, hormone replacement therapy	No specific intervention, sRAGE/AGE breakers	No specific intervention, gene therapy	Pain medication, anti-inflammatory drugs

Table 1.1 Differentiation of clinical osteoarthritis phenotypes. AGE, advanced glycation endproducts; sRAGE, soluble receptor for advanced glycation endproducts. Data from Bijlsma et al [15]. © 2011, reproduced with permission from Elsevier.

The evolution of osteoarthritis management

Pain is the first and primary osteoarthritis symptom that drives patients to see their doctor[15]. While willow extract was used in ancient times for pain control, it was not until the 18th century when modern accounts of its usage began to appear[26]. The isolation and then synthetic production of the active constituents led to the introduction of aspirin (acetylsalicylic acid) by Bayer in 1899[27], which was followed by their development of paracetamol[26]. Later, nonsteroidal anti-inflammatory drugs (NSAIDs) were developed[26]; however, it was only with the understanding of the mechanism of action of NSAIDs in the 1970s that the targeting of just the cyclooxygenase (COX)-2 enzyme, with the consequent reduction in gastrointestinal events associated with the COX-1 enzyme, was possible[26]. While the use of opioids for osteoarthritis management has increased, there is a lack of evidence of the long-term safety and efficacy of the weaker forms of these drugs in patients with osteoarthritis[15].

Symptomatic slow-acting drugs are also sometimes used for osteoarthritis treatment, including glucosamine sulphate, chondroitin sulphate, hyaluronic acid, diacerhein and avocado soybean unsaponifiable. However, the effectiveness of many of these therapies remains a matter of debate[15]. Interestingly, the usage of more antiquated methods of pain control are being investigated for the management of knee osteoarthritis. Leech therapy was shown to significantly improve self-reported pain scores within 24 hours, with improvements sustained at 4 weeks (Figure 1.4)[28].

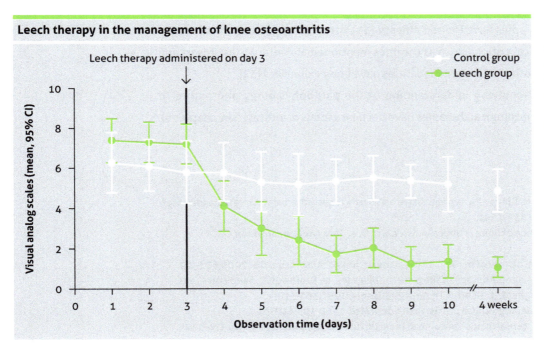

Leech therapy in the management of knee osteoarthritis

Figure 1.4 Leech therapy in the management of knee osteoarthritis. Pain was measured on visual analogue scales. Pain scores improved from 7.4 at baseline to 1.3 at Day 10 ($P<0.001$) and remained stable at 4-week follow-up with a score of 1.0. In the control group, the equivalent scores were 6.3, 5.2 and 4.8. CI, confidence interval. Reproduced with permission from Michalsen et al [28].

Joint replacement surgery has been available for the hip for 40 years and knee replacement for around 30 years. The number of knee replacements is increasing at a rate greater than that of hip replacements, such that the demand for the two procedures is now about equal[29]. Other surgical interventions include arthroscopy, osteotomy, joint fusion, joint distraction and surgical lavage and debridement, although the latter procedure is not advised[15].

While there is currently no cure for osteoarthritis, current management strategies, which advocate a comprehensive treatment plan based on meeting established clinical radiographical criteria (Table 1.2), aim to primarily reduce pain and improve joint function through targeted symptom relief [15,30]. Alongside self-management and educational programs and exercise and assistive devices, pharmacologic therapy is one of the primary tools in the armamentarium of the physician managing osteoarthritis. Drugs used to treat osteoarthritis include:

- simple analgesics;
- NSAIDs;
- intra-articular therapies;
- supplements or alternative therapy; and
- disease modification therapy.

American College of Rheumatology radiological and clinical criteria for knee osteoarthritis	
Knee (clinical)	Knee (clinical and radiographic)
Osteoarthritis if 1, 2, 3, 4 or 1, 2, 5 or 1, 4, 5 are present:	*Osteoarthritis if 1, 2 or 1, 3, 5, 6 or 1, 4, 5, 6 are present:*
1. Knee pain for most days of previous month	1. Knee pain for most days of previous month
2. Crepitus on active joint motion	2. Osteophytes at joint margins on radiographs
3. Morning stiffness lasting 30 min or less	3. Synovial fluid typical of OA (laboratory)
4. Age 38 years or older	4. Age 40 years or older
5. Bony enlargement of the knee on examination	5. Crepitus on active joint motion
	6. Morning stiffness lasting 30 min or less

Table 1.2 American College of Rheumatology radiological and clinical criteria for knee osteoarthritis. Table from Bijlsma et al [15]. © 2011, reproduced with permission from Elsevier.

However, current drug therapies have limited efficacy [31], often leaving patients with a substantial pain burden. Surgical options, such as the ones mentioned above, are a last-resort and should be used only when other treatment modalities have been exhausted [32].

Building on our ever-evolving understanding of the pathophysiology and nature of osteoarthritis, novel pharmacological therapies have become a focus of interest (see chapter 6).

References

1   Conaghan PG, Vanharanta H, Dieppe PA. Is progressive osteoarthritis an atheromatous vascular disease? *Ann Rheum Dis.* 2005;64:1539-1541.
2   Neogi T. Clinical significance of bone changes in osteoarthritis. *Ther Adv Musculoskelet Dis.* 2012;4:259-267.
3   Dequeker J, Luyten FP. The history of osteoarthritis-osteoarthrosis. *Ann Rheum Dis.* 2008;67:5-10.
4   Bourke J. A review of the paleopathology of the arthritic diseases. In: Brothwell D, Sandison A, eds. *Diseases in Antique.* Springfield, IL: Charles Thomas Publishers; 1967:361-370.
5   Karsh R, McCarthy J. Archaeology and arthritis. *Arch Intern Med.* 1960;105:640-644.
6   Benedek TG. When did "osteo-arthritis" become osteoarthritis? *J Rheumatol.* 1999;26:1374-1376.
7   Heberden W. *Commentaries on the History and Cure of Diseases.* London, UK: T. Payne; 1802.
8   Brodie BC. *Pathological and Surgical Observations on the Diseases of the Joints.* 2nd ed. London, UK: Longman, Hurst, Rees, Orne and Brown; 1822.
9   Smith R. Malum coxae senilis. *Dublin J Med Chem Sci.* 1835;6:205.
10 Kellgren JH, Moore R. Generalized osteoarthritis and Heberden's nodes. *Br Med J.* 1952;1:181-187.
11 Kellgren JH, Lawrence JS. Radiological assessment of osteo-arthrosis. *Ann Rheum Dis.* 1957;16:494-502.

12 van Saase JL, van Romunde LK, Cats A, Vandenbroucke JP, Valkenburg HA. Epidemiology of osteoarthritis: Zoetermeer survey. Comparison of radiological osteoarthritis in a Dutch population with that in 10 other populations. *Ann Rheum Dis.* 1989;48:271-280.

13 Benedek TG. A history of the understanding of cartilage. *Osteoarthr Cartilage.* 2006;14:203-209.

14 Slack H. Some notes on the composition and metabolism of connective tissue. *Am J Med.* 1959;26:113-124.

15 Bijlsma JWJ, Berenbaum F, Lafeber FPJG. Osteoarthritis: an update with relevance for clinical practice. *Lancet.* 2011;377:2115-2126.

16 Sellam J, Berenbaum F. The role of synovitis in pathophysiology and clinical symptoms of osteoarthritis. *Nat Rev Rheumatol.* 2010;6:625-635.

17 Rogers J, Shepstone L, Dieppe P. Is osteoarthritis a systemic disorder of bone? *Arthritis Rheum.* 2004;50:452-457.

18 Rogers J, Shepstone L, Dieppe P. Bone formers: osteophyte and enthesophyte formation are positively associated. *Ann Rheum Dis.* 1997;56:85-90.

19 Hasegawa A, Otsuki S, Pauli C, et al. Anterior cruciate ligament changes in the human knee joint in aging and osteoarthritis. *Arthritis Rheum.* 2012;64:696-704.

20 Felson DT, Chaisson CE, Hill CL, et al. The association of bone marrow lesions with pain in knee osteoarthritis. *Ann Intern Med.* 2001;134:541-549.

21 Burr DB, Gallant MA. Bone remodelling in osteoarthritis. *Nat Rev Rheumatol.* 2012;8:665-673.

22 Waldron HA. Prevalence and distribution of osteoarthritis in a population from Georgian and early Victorian London. *Ann Rheum Dis.* 1991;50:301-307.

23 Waldron HA. Association between osteoarthritis of the hand and knee in a population of skeletons from London. *Ann Rheum Dis.* 1997;56:116-118.

24 Cushnaghan J, Dieppe P. Study of 500 patients with limb joint osteoarthritis. I. Analysis by age, sex, and distribution of symptomatic joint sites. *Ann Rheum Dis.* 1991;50:8-13.

25 Hirsch R, Lethbridge-Cejku M, Scott WW Jr, et al. Association of hand and knee osteoarthritis: evidence for a polyarticular disease subset. *Ann Rheum Dis.* 1996;55:25-29.

26 Appelboom T. Arthropathy in art and the history of pain management—through the centuries to cyclooxygenase-2 inhibitors. *Rheumatology (Oxford).* 2002;41(suppl 1):28-34.

27 Mann R. The history of non-steroidal anti-Inflammatory agents. In: Mann R, ed. *The History of the Management of Pain: From Early Principles to Present Practice.* Carnforth, UK: Parthenon Publishing Group; 1988:77-119.

28 Michalsen A, Moebus S, Spahn G, Esch T, Langhorst J, Dobos GJ. Leech therapy for symptomatic treatment of knee osteoarthritis: results and implications of a pilot study. *Altern Ther Health Med.* 2002;8:84-88.

29 Dubey S, Adebajo AO. Historical and current perspectives on management of osteoarthritis and rheumatoid arthritis. In: Reid DM, Miller CG, eds. *Clinical Trials in Rheumatoid Arthritis and Osteoarthritis.* London, UK: Springer-Verlag London Limited; 2008:5-36.

30 Hunter DJ, Lo GH. The management of osteoarthritis: an overview and call to appropriate conservative treatment. *Rheum Dis Clin North Am.* 2008;34:689-712.

31 Zhang W, Nuki G, Moskowitz RW, et al. OARSI recommendations for the management of hip and knee osteoarthritis: Part III: changes in evidence following systematic cumulative update of research published through January 2009. *Osteoarthritis Cartilage.* 2010;18:476-499.

32 Richmond JC. Surgery for osteoarthritis of the knee. *Rheum Dis Clin North Am.* 2008;34:815-825.

Chapter 2
Epidemiology of osteoarthritis

Cyrus Cooper, M. Kassim Javaid and Nigel Arden

Definition of osteoarthritis

" *A group of overlapping disorders with different aetiologies but similar biologic, morphologic and clinical outcomes. The disease processes affect articular cartilage, subchondral bone, synovium, capsule and ligaments. Ultimately, cartilage degenerates with fibrillation, fissures, ulceration and full thickness loss of joint surface.* "

Nigel Arden

This definition is itself developed from one coined by the Diagnostic and Therapeutic Criteria Committee of the American Rheumatism Association for the development of criteria for classifying and reporting osteoarthritis in 1986 [1]. It also made the distinction between subclinical, non-symptomatic defects in articular cartilage, which is poorly innervated, and the clinical syndrome, which includes pain, that may develop from such defects [1].

" *Knee osteoarthritis is characterised clinically by usage-related pain and/or functional limitation. It is a common complex joint disorder showing focal cartilage loss, new bone formation and involvement of all joint tissues. Structural tissue changes are mirrored in classical radiographic features.* "

The European League Against Rheumatism

" *A heterogeneous group of conditions that lead to joint symptoms and signs which are associated with defective integrity of articular cartilage, in addition to related changes in the underlying bone at the joint margins.* "

American College of Rheumatology

A specific definition of knee osteoarthritis was developed in 2010 for the European League Against Rheumatism (EULAR) evidence-based recommendations for the diagnosis of knee osteoarthritis [2]. The EULAR recommendations, which emphasise that knee osteoarthritis may associate with osteoarthritis at other joints due to shared genetic and constitutional risk symptoms, also highlight that the definition of knee osteoarthritis may change based on the different levels of care needed and the clinical requirements [2].

This publication has been made possible through an educational grant from SERVIER.

N. Arden et al., *Atlas of Osteoarthritis*, DOI 10.1007/978-1-910315-16-3_2,
© Springer Healthcare 2014

Classification of osteoarthritis

In 1957, Kellgren and Lawrence developed a classification system that sets out a series of radio-logical features that are considered evidence of osteoarthritis, and divides the disease into five grades (Figure 2.1) [3]:

- 0 – None
- 1 – Doubtful
- 2 – Minimal
- 3 – Moderate
- 4 – Severe

Grade 0 indicates a definite absence of osteoarthritis changes on a single anteroposterior X-ray, while grade 2 represents definite osteoarthritis, albeit of minimal severity [3]. Although the system is widely used, it has limitations, particularly when assessing individual radiographic features.

Radiographic classification of osteoarthritis

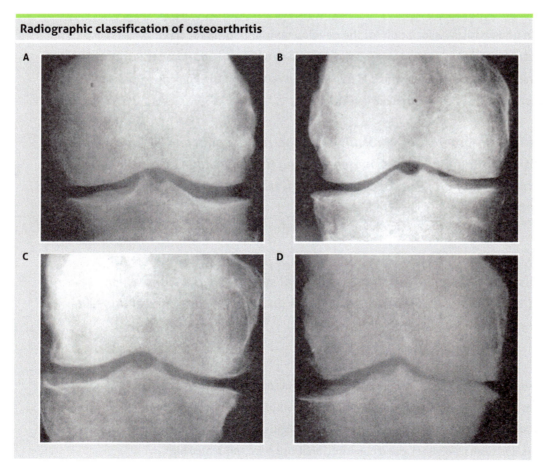

Figure 2.1 Radiographic classification of osteoarthritis.
A, Grade 1: doubtful joint space narrowing (JSN) and possible osteophytic lipping.
B, Grade 2: definite osteophytes and possible JSN.
C, Grade 3: moderate multiple osteophytes, definite JSN, some sclerosis, possible bone end deformity.
D, Grade 4: large osteophytes, marked JSN, severe sclerosis definite deformity of bone ends. Image from Kellgren & Lawrence [3]. © 1957, reproduced with permission from BMJ Publishing Group Ltd.

The radiological features of knee osteoarthritis were refined by the Osteoarthritis Research Society International in 2007 [4], and divided into: the presence of marginal osteophytes in the medial femoral condyle, medial tibial plateau, lateral femoral condyle and lateral tibial plateau (Figure 2.2) [5] and joint space narrowing (JSN) of the medial compartment and lateral compartment. Each of these are graded for degree of change:

- 0 – Normal
- 1 – Mild change
- 2 – Moderate change
- 3 – Severe change

Femoral osteophytes

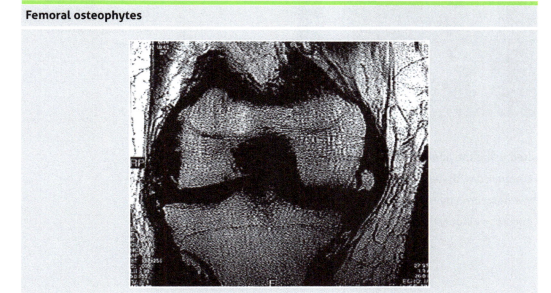

Figure 2.2 Femoral osteophytes. This coronal magnetic resonance image of an osteoarthritis knee is a T1-weighted spin-echo image that shows femoral osteophytes on the medial and lateral aspects of the joint. The bright signal within the osteophytes is produced by marrow fat. Reproduced with permission from Myers [5].

Recently, a Delphi exercise was undertaken to develop definitions of osteoarthritis on magnetic resonance imaging (MRI), which suggested that, while MRI changes of osteoarthritis may occur in the absence of radiographic findings, MRI changes in isolation and single MRI changes, are not diagnostic of osteoarthritis [6]. Nevertheless, a definition of tibiofemoral osteoarthritis on MRI was developed (Figure 2.3, see page 22) [7], which was either the presence of two features from group A, or one group A feature plus at least two group B features, where:

- Group A, after exclusion of joint trauma within the last 6 months and exclusion of inflammatory arthritis:
  - Definite osteophyte formation
  - Full thickness cartilage loss
- Group B:
  - Subchondral bone marrow lesion or cyst not associated with meniscal or ligamentous attachments
  - Meniscal subluxation, maceration or degenerative (horizontal) tear
  - Partial thickness cartilage loss (where full thickness loss is not present)
  - Bone attrition

Magnetic resonance imaging of the knee: remodelling and sclerosis

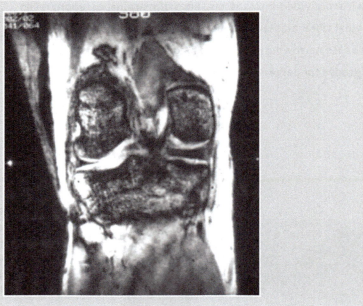

Figure 2.3 Magnetic resonance imaging of the knee: remodelling and sclerosis. This magnetic resonance image reveals considerable subchondral bone remodelling and sclerosis. Posteriorly, the cartilage of the lateral compartment is thickened with thinning and irregular cartilage in the medial compartment. Reproduced with permission from Altman [7].

A composite model was created using the above features to assess the ability of MRI to detect radiographic osteoarthritis compared with Kellgren and Lawrence (KL) grade 2, which yielded a C statistic of 0.59, which was described by the authors as "disappointing" [6]. Nevertheless, MRI retains the potential to diagnose osteoarthritis earlier than the current reference standard of radiography [6].

Prevalence and incidence of osteoarthritis

The prevalence of osteoarthritis has been assessed in a number of studies spanning several decades. van Saase et al examined the prevalence of mild and severe radiological osteoarthritis in a single Dutch village, finding that increased radiological osteoarthritis is strongly linked to age, regardless of whether small or large weight-bearing joints are considered, and holds for both men and women (Figure 2.4) [8].

The highest prevalence for osteoarthritis is seen in the cervical spine, the lumbar spine and the distal interphalangeal joints (DIP) [8]. Severe radiological osteoarthritis is uncommon under age 45 years, and the prevalence does not exceed 20% in the elderly aside from in the cervical and lumbar spine and DIP and, in women, the joints of the hands and the knees [8]. Significant sex differences are seen in the knees, in the hips among those aged at least 65 years and in the DIP of the hands [8]. Comparison with other populations shows that, although there are substantial differences between populations for individual joints, the slope of the majority of lines is similar for individual and groups of joints, with no one population having a low or high prevalence of osteoarthritis for all joints [8].

Epidemiology of osteoarthritis

Prevalence of osteoarthritis

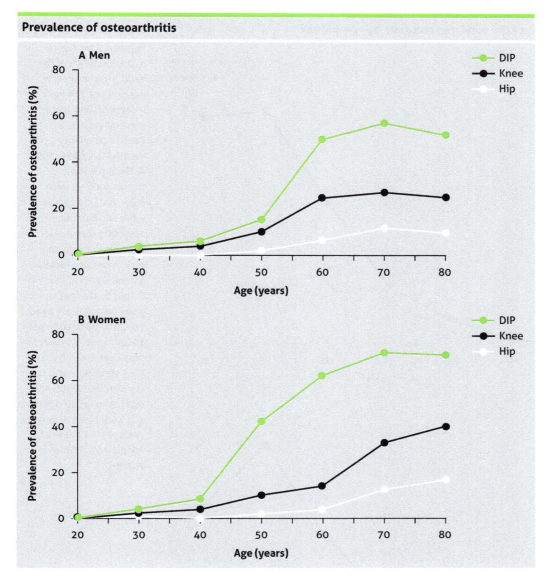

Figure 2.4 Prevalence of osteoarthritis. A random sample of a Dutch village demonstrated the high prevalence of radiological osteoarthritis, which increases progressively with age. Mild radiological osteoarthritis is more prevalent in women (**B**) than in men (**A**), while severe radiological osteoarthritis is substantially more prevalent in women. DIP, distal interphalangeal joints. Data from van Saase et al [8]. © 1989, reproduced with permission from BMJ Publishing Group Ltd.

The incidence of osteoarthritis increases with age, and women have higher incidences than men, especially after age 50 (Figure 2.5, see page 24) [9]. The incidence of knee osteoarthritis is twice that of hand or hip osteoarthritis, and the female:male sex ratio for hand, hip and knee osteoarthritis is approximately 2:1. The trend of increasing osteoarthritis incidence continues until age 80 after which there is a levelling off or decline in the rates for all joints, which may be linked to sedentary activity in older age groups [9].

The lifetime risk of undergoing total hip replacement (THR) or total knee replacement (TKR) is lower than that of developing symptomatic knee or hip osteoarthritis [10]. The mortality-adjusted lifetime risk of undergoing THR at age 50 years is estimated, using 2005 data, at 11.6% for women and 7.1% for men, while the risks of undergoing TKR are 10.8% and 8.1%, respectively [10]. The risk decreases with increasing age for THR and TKR in both men and women, such that, at 80 years of age, the lifetime risk of THR is 3.8% for women and 2.7% for men, while that for TKR is 3.3% and 2.7%, respectively [10].

Incidence of osteoarthritis of the hand, hip and knee by age and sex

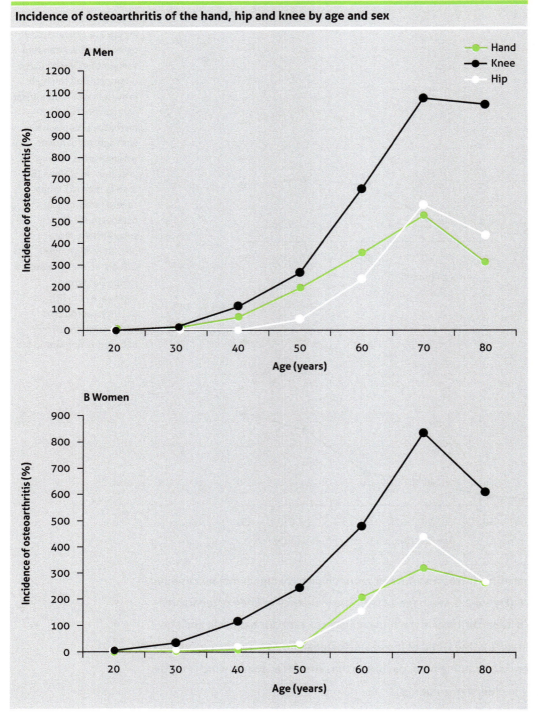

Figure 2.5 Incidence of osteoarthritis of the hand, hip and knee by age and sex. The data represents incidence in members of the Fallon Community Health Plan, 1991–1992. **A**, The equivalent figures for men were 5 per 100,000 person-years and 619 per 100,000 person-years. **B**, Among women, the incidence rates for knee osteoarthritis ranged from 0 per 100,000 person-years among those aged 20–29 years to 1082 per 100,000 person-years for those aged 70–79 years. The overall age- and sex-standardised incidence rate for knee osteoarthritis was 240/100,000 person-years (95% CI 218–262). Adapted from Oliveria et al [9].

Interestingly, the rates of primary TKR have increased substantially over the last two decades, much more so than for THR (Figure 2.6) [11]. This may reflect the more recent maturation of TKR as an efficacious treatment for osteoarthritis, or be because the number TKRs performed each year is below that which would be appropriate for the burden of osteoarthritis of the knee [11].

Trends in primary total knee replacement rates

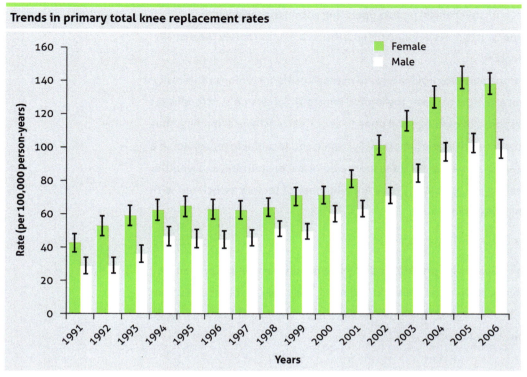

Figure 2.6 Trends in primary total knee replacement rates. During the study period (1991–2006), the estimated age-standardised rates of primary total knee replacement (TKR) increased from 42.5 (95% CI 37.0–48.0) to 138.7 (95% CI 132.3–145.0) in women and from 28.7 (95% CI 23.9–33.6) to 99.4 (95% CI 93.9–104.8) in men. Interestingly, there was a marked plateau in TKR rates from the mid-1990s, followed by a sharp rise from 2000. Data from Culliford et al [11]. © 2012, reproduced with permission from The British Editorial Society of Bone and Joint Surgery.

Aetiology and risk factors

In order to understand the influence that risks factors for osteoarthritis have on the pathogenesis, a conceptual framework for the disease has been developed in recent years that consists of the following tenets (Figure 2.7) [12–18]:

Risk factors for osteoarthritis

Systemic factors:
1. *Age*
2. *Gender*
3. *Ethnic*
4. Hormonal status
5. Genetic factors
6. Bone density
7. Nutritional factors (vitamin C and D are protective)
8. Inflammation

Local joint factors:
1. Previous damage
2. Muscle weakness
3. Joint deformity/ incongruity
4. Ligamentous laxity

Extrinsic factors acting on joints:
1. *Obesity*
2. Specific injurious activities:
   - Sport and physical activities (excess)
   - Occupational factors (eg, farming)

Susceptibility to osteoarthritis or to its progression

Figure 2.7 Risk factors for osteoarthritis. Several systemic factors have been identified as risk factors for knee osteoarthritis, which may act by increasing the susceptibility of joints to injury, via direct damage to joint tissues, or by impairing the repair process in damaged joint tissue. Local biomechanical factors are, in contrast, believed primarily to determine the exposure of individual joints to injury and to excess loading that leads to joint degeneration. Adapted from [16–18].

- Cartilage, bone, muscles, ligaments and other joint tissues and structures function as a biomechanical organ system that maintains proper movement and prevents excessive joint loading;
- Systemic factors that increase overall susceptibility to joint degeneration, and local biomechanical factors that impair the optimal functioning of a joint both play an important role in determining the risk of developing osteoarthritis; and

- Systemic factors interact with mechanical factors operating within the local joint environment to determine which joints develop osteoarthritis and how rapidly the disease progresses in an affected joint.

It is suggested that several of the pathological features of osteoarthritis, including proliferative bone changes, may represent attempts to repair the injured joint [19]. For example, osteophytes may arise from a reactive response of cartilage and bone to abnormal mechanical loading, thus reducing instability to protect the damaged joint [12]. Systemic and local factors may act in a joint-specific manner to determine whether such a response is normal or aberrant, and whether it succeeds or fails in protecting the joint [12]. There are a number of factors associated with osteoarthritis of the knee, hip and hand.

Age

The age-related increases in osteoarthritis prevalence and incidence are particularly pronounced in the commonly affected joints, such as the knee, hip and hand. It is thought that the relationship between age and the risk of osteoarthritis is mediated by age-related increases in a range of systemic and biomechanical risk factors [12].

Sex

Female gender amplifies the age-related increase in osteoarthritis risk in the hands and knees, as well as osteoarthritis in multiple joints, such that, after 50 years of age, the prevalence and incidence is significantly greater in women than men [9,20]. While hip osteoarthritis appears to progress more rapidly in women [21,22], there appears to be no gender impact on knee [23,24], or hand osteoarthritis progression [12].

Ethnicity

The prevalence of osteoarthritis and patterns of affected joints vary among racial and ethnic groups [25]. Osteoarthritis is, in general, more prevalent in Europe and the USA than other parts of the world [26]. Osteoarthritis of the knee is more common in African-American women than white women [27], but that is not the case for the hip [28]. Osteoarthritis of the hip is more common in European whites than in Jamaican blacks [29], African blacks [30] or Chinese [31]. The Beijing Osteoarthritis Study indicated that hip and hand osteoarthritis was less frequent among Chinese than in whites in the Framingham Study, although the prevalence of radiographic and symptomatic knee osteoarthritis was significantly higher in Chinese women than in white women [32,33].

Menopause

As the increase in the age-related rise in osteoarthritis occurs following menopause, it would suggest that sex hormones, particularly oestrogen deficiency, play a role in the systemic predisposition to osteoarthritis [12]. While many studies have looked at the possibility of lowering osteoarthritis risk through oestrogen use, any associations may be misleading, as oestrogen use is linked to a healthy lifestyle and osteoporosis, which lowers the risk of osteoarthritis [12].

Genetic factors

Genetic vulnerability appears to account for approximately half the variability of susceptibility to hand, hip and knee osteoarthritis in women [34–40] and men [38,39]. These studies suggest that not only are multiple genes likely to be involved in osteoarthritis susceptibility but also that environmental factors have an important role in progression [12]. The search for candidate genes has focused on genes encoding type II collagen (the primary collagen in articular cartilage), structural proteins of the extracellular cartilage matrix, the vitamin D and oestrogen receptor genes, as well as encoding bone and cartilage growth factors [41].

Obesity

Obesity is one of the most well-established and strongest risk factors for knee osteoarthritis [13], and precedes the development of knee osteoarthritis by many years [42–44]. In addition, obesity accelerates the progression of knee osteoarthritis [45,46]. The primary mechanism for the impact of obesity of knee osteoarthritis is likely to be excess weight on overloading of the joints during weight-bearing activities, leading to breakdown of cartilage and damage to ligaments and other support structures [12]. Metabolic factors, such as circulating adipocytokines, adiposity-linked glucose and lipid abnormalities and chronic inflammation, may also play a role in the pathogenesis of osteoarthritis [12].

Mechanical and occupational factors and trauma

Acute knee injuries, including meniscal and cruciate ligament tears in the knee, fractures and dislocations [12], substantially increase the risk of any subsequent osteoarthritis, as well that of more severe disease [45]. In addition, the risk of osteoarthritis is increased by weekly participation in sports for a decade or longer after leaving school [44]. Specifically, repetitive and excessive joint loading due to specific physical activities increases the risk of developing osteoarthritis in the stressed joints [12].

Congenital and developmental diseases

The risk of developing osteoarthritis is substantially increased as a result of congenital abnormalities that result in abnormal load distributions within the joint [47]. As the mechanical alignment of the knee, as determined by the hip/knee/ankle angle, is an important determinant of load distribution of the knee during ambulation [48], varus and valgus malalignment are found with a high frequency in knees with evidence of osteoarthritis involvement of the medial and lateral components, respectively [49]. Osteoarthritic knees with varus malalignment have a three- to fourfold increased risk of further joint space narrowing in the medial compartment, which is similar to the increased risk of further lateral compartment joint space narrowing in osteoarthritis knees with valgus malalignment [50]. Discoveries about the pathophysiology of the disease have led to a potential division of the disease into distinct phenotypes (see Table 1.1) [51]. In addition to improving our understanding of the disease, classifying the different clinical and structural phenotypes of osteoarthritis allows for more direct targeting of treatments, depending on where the predominate structural changes are, eg, cartilage, bone or synovial tissue. However, there is currently no consensus on the subgrouping of osteoarthritis into these phenotypes [51].

Disease course and determinants of osteoarthritis progression

There are a number of biomarkers under investigation for the assessment of osteoarthritis progression, as the identification of rapid progressors would assist in the development and targeting of therapies. Imaging technologies such as MRI appear promising in the assessment of disease progression, and combining biochemical and MRI-based biomarkers may offer effective diagnostic and prognostic tools for identifying osteoarthritis patients at high risk of progression (Figure 2.8) [52]. While cartilage roughness is a good diagnostic marker, with an area under the receiver operating characteristics curve (AUC) of 0.80, and cartilage homogeneity performs well as a prognostic marker, with an AUC of 0.71, an aggregate marker of cartilage matrix breakdown and cartilage volume, thickness, area, congruity, roughness and homogeneity performs well both diagnostically and prognostically, at respective AUCs of 0.84 and 0.77 [52].

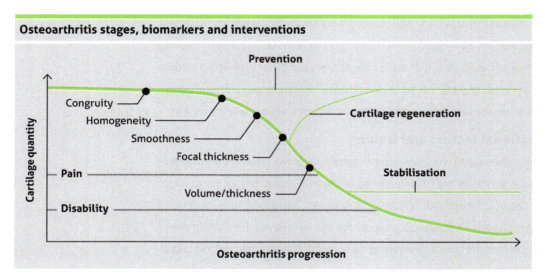

Osteoarthritis stages, biomarkers and interventions

Figure 2.8 Osteoarthritis stages, biomarkers and interventions. Figure courtesy of Dr C Cooper.

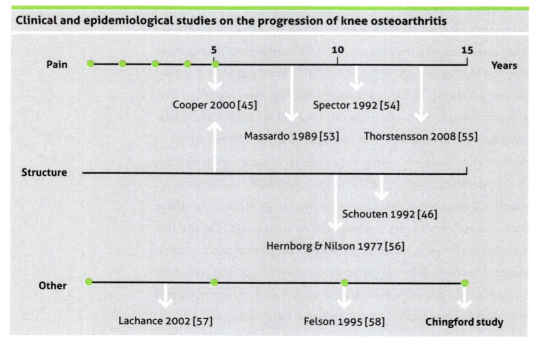

Clinical and epidemiological studies on the progression of knee osteoarthritis

Figure 2.9 Clinical and epidemiological studies on the progression of knee osteoarthritis. Circles represent the timings of the visits for the Chingford study. Figure courtesy of Dr K Leyland. Data from [45,46,53–58].

There have been a number of studies that have examined the progression of osteoarthritis over follow-up periods of up to 15 years, including the recently published Chingford study (Figure 2.9) [45,46,53–58].

The evolution of knee osteoarthritis is slow, it typically takes several years and can remain stable for several years [21]. Radiographic deterioration is seen in a third to two-thirds of osteoarthritis patients and radiographic improvement is unusual (Table 2.1) [45,46,53,54,59–65].

Natural history of knee osteoarthritis

Study	N	Measure	Years	Deterioration (%)
Hernborg & Nilson (1977) [56]	94	C	15	55
		R	15	56
Danielsson (1970) [59]	106	R	15	33
Massardo (1989) [53]	31	R	8	42
Dougados (1992) [60]	353	C	1	28
		R	1	29
Schouten (1992) [46]	142	R	12	34
Spector (1992) [54]	63	R	11	33
Spector (1994) [61]	58	R	2	22
Ledingham (1995) [62]	350	R	2	72
McAlindon (1999) [63]	470	R	4	11
Cooper et al (2000) [45]	354	R	5	22
Felson (2004) [64]	323	R	2.5	28

Table 2.1 Natural history of knee osteoarthritis. C, Clinical; R, Radiographic. Table adapted with permission from Dennison & Cooper [65]. Data from [45,46,53,54,59–64].

Odds ratio of incidence and progression of knee osteoarthritis

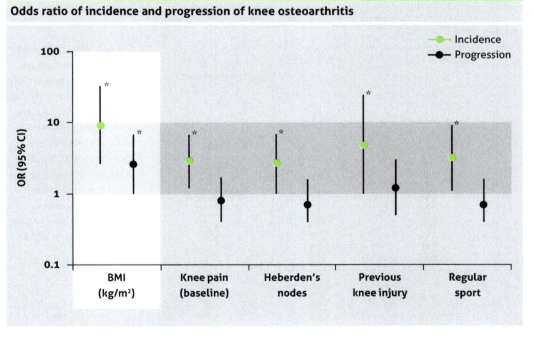

Figure 2.10 Odds ratio of incidence and progression of knee osteoarthritis. The odds ratio (OR) was calculated over 5 years among patients with Kellgren and Lawrence grade 1+ disease. OR are adjusted for age and sex in all cases. In addition, OR for BMI, knee pain and Heberden's nodes are mutually adjusted. OR for knee injury and sports participation are adjusted for age, sex, BMI, knee pain and Heberden's nodes. Obesity was a strong predictor of incidence knee osteoarthritis (P<0.001) and a significant predictor of progression (P<0.05). BMI, Body mass index; CI, confidence interval. *Significant increase in risk. Data from Cooper et al [45].

While there are several factors significantly associated with the incidence of osteoarthritis, only obesity is significantly individually linked to the progression of grade 1+ disease (Figure 2.10) [45]. In addition, the coexistence of Heberden's nodes with knee osteoarthritis increases the risk of knee deterioration by almost sixfold [21].

The Chingford study looked at the progression of individual KL grades over 15 years (Table 2.2) [66], which revealed that approximately half of knees had a KL grade of 0 throughout, while two-fifths worsened by at least one grade. Knees with baseline KL grade 1 had a higher percentage of progression, at almost three-quarters, than knees with any other KL grade at baseline. Less than 2% of knees were scored as having regressed to a lower KL grade by year 15 [43].

Progression of individual Kellgren and Lawrence grades over 15 years

Baseline Kellgren and Lawrence grade	N	Year 15 Kellgren and Lawrence grade					
		0	1	2	3	4	5
0	905	60.1% (548)	9.9% (90)	15.7% (142)	12.5% (113)	0.1% (1)	1.2% (11)
1	57	19.3% (11)	5.3% (3)	40.4% (23)	29.8% (17)	0.0% (0)	5.3% (3)
2	60	0 (0.0%)	1.7% (1)	50.0% (30)	41.7% (25)	0.0% (0)	6.7% (4)
3	26	0.0% (0)	3.8% (1)	15.4% (4)	65.4% (17)	11.5% (3)	3.8% (1)

Table 2.2 Progression of individual Kellgren and Lawrence grades over 15 years. Data from Leyland et al [66].

The prevalence of long-term knee pain is dependent on whether there was any pain at baseline (Figure 2.11) [67]. The presence of knee osteoarthritis increases the risk of persistent pain by 3.70-fold, while reported knee injury increases the risk of persistent pain 4.13-fold and intermittent pain 4.25-fold [44]. Interestingly, there is a discrepancy between the presence of radiographic osteoarthritis and corresponding pain, which may be due to KL grade being a predictor only of persistent, and not intermittent pain.

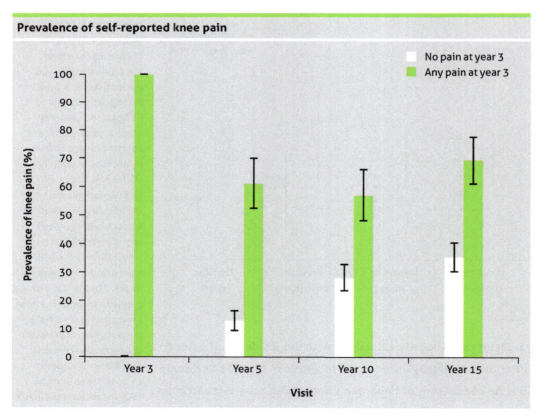

Prevalence of self-reported knee pain

Figure 2.11 Prevalence of self-reported knee pain. Bars show the means with 95% confidence intervals. Individuals without knee pain at baseline (year 3) had an increase in pain prevalence with duration of follow-up, such that, at year 15, the prevalence was 35.2% for those reporting any days of pain. Data from Soni et al [67].

Another important consideration in the assessment of osteoarthritis is the presence of comorbidities. It is estimated that older osteoarthritis patients have an average of 8.7 chronic medical diseases [68]. The three most common comorbidities are obesity, hypertension and high cholesterol levels (Figure 2.12) [69].

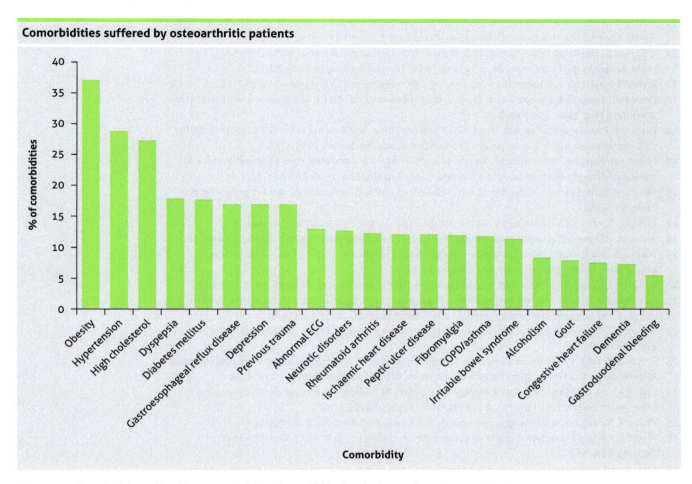

Comorbidities suffered by osteoarthritic patients

Figure 2.12 Comorbidities suffered by osteoarthritic patients. COPD, chronic obstructive pulmonary disorder; ECG, electrocardiography. Data from Datamonitor [69].

References

1   Altman R, Asch E, Bloch D, et al. Development of criteria for the classification and reporting of osteoarthritis. Classification of osteoarthritis of the knee. Diagnostic and therapeutic criteria committee of the American Rheumatism Association. *Arthritis Rheum.* 1986;29:1039-1049.
2   Zhang W, Doherty M, Peat G, et al. EULAR evidence-based recommendations for the diagnosis of knee osteoarthritis. *Ann Rheum Dis.* 2010;69:483-489.
3   Kellgren J, Lawrence J. Radiological assessment of osteo-arthrosis. *Ann Rheum Dis.* 1957;16:494-502.
4   Altman R, Gold G. Atlas of individual radiographic features in osteoarthritis, revised. *Osteo Cart.* 2007;15 Suppl A:A1-56.
5   Myers S. Osteoarthritis and crystal-associated synovitis. In: Hunder G, ed. *Atlas of Rheumatology.* 4th ed. Philadelphia: Current Medicine Group; 2005:54-64.
6   Hunter D, Arden N, Conaghan P, et al. Definition of osteoarthritis on MRI: results of a Delphi exercise. *Osteo Cart.* 2011;19:963-969.
7   Altman R. Osteoarthritis in the elderly population. In: Nakasato Y, Yung R, eds. *Geriatric Rheumatology. A Comprehensive Approach.* New York: Springer; 2011:187-196.

8   van Saase JL, Van Romunde LK, Cats A, Vandenbroucke J, Valkenburg H. Epidemiology of osteoarthritis: Zoetermeer survey. Comparison of radiological osteoarthritis in a Dutch population with that in 10 other populations. *Ann Rheum Dis*. 1989;48:271-280.

9   Oliveria S, Felson D, Reed J, Cirillo P, Walker A. Incidence of symptomatic hand, hip, and knee osteoarthritis among patients in a health maintenance organization. *Arthritis Rheum*. 1995;38:1134-1141.

10   Culliford D, Maskell J, Kiran A, et al. The lifetime risk of total hip and knee arthroplasty: results from the UK General Practice Research Database. *Osteo Cart*. 2012;20:519-524.

11   Culliford D, Maskell J, Beard D, Murray D, Price A, Arden N. Temporal trends in hip and knee replacement in the United Kingdom: 1991 to 2006. *J Bone Joint Surg Br*. 2010;92:130-135.

12   Arden N, Nevitt M. Osteoarthritis: Epidemiology. *Best Pract Res Clin Rheumatol*. 2006;20:3-25.

13   Felson D, Lawrence R, Dieppe P, et al. Osteoarthritis: new insights. Part 1: The disease and its risk factors. *Ann Intern Med*. 2000;133:635-646.

14   Dieppe P. The classification and diagnosis of osteoarthritis. In: Kuettner K, Vm G, eds. *Osteoarthritic Disorders*. Rosemont, IL: American Academy of Orthopedic Surgeons; 1995:5-12.

15   Sharma H, Hanna A, Titterington L, Stephens R. Effect of MAK-4 and MAK-5 on endothelial cell and soyabean lipoxygenase-induced LDL oxidation. *Adv Exp Med Biol*. 1994;366:441-443.

16   Garstand S. Osteoarthritis: epidemiology, risk factors and pathophysiology. *Am J Phys Med Rehabil*. 2006;85: S2-S11.

17   Zhang Y, Jordan J. Epidemiology of osteoarthritis. *Clin Geriatr Med*. 2010;26:355-369.

18   Woolf A, Pfleger B. Burden of major musculoskeletal conditions. *WHO Bulletin*. 2003;81:646-656.

19   Dieppe P. Subchondral bone should be the main target for the treatment of pain and disease progression in osteoarthritis. *Osteo Cart*. 1999;7:325-326.

20   Kellgren J, Moore R. Generalized osteoarthritis and Heberden's nodes. *Br Med J*. 1952;1:181-187.

21   Dougados M, Gueguen A, Nguyen M, et al. Radiological progression of hip osteoarthritis: definition, risk factors and correlations with clinical status. *Ann Rheum Dis*. 1996;55:356-362.

22   Loeser R, Shakoor N. Aging or osteoarthritis: which is the problem? *Rheum Dis Clin North Am*. 2003;29:653-673.

23   Felson D, Naimark A, Anderson J, Kazis L, Castelli W, Meenan R. The prevalence of knee osteoarthritis in the elderly. The Framingham osteoarthritis study. *Arthritis Rheum*. 1987;30:914-918.

24   Ledingham J, Dawson S, Preston B, Milligan G, Doherty M. Radiographic progression of hospital referred osteoarthritis of the hip. *Ann Rheum Dis*. 1993;52(4):263-267.

25   Zhang Y, Jordan J. Epidemiology of osteoarthritis. *Clin Geriatr Med*. 2010;26:355-369.

26   Woolf A, Pfleger B. Burden of major musculoskeletal conditions. *Bull World Health Organ*. 2003;81:646-656.

27   Anderson J, Felson D. Factors associated with osteoarthritis of the knee in the first national Health and Nutrition Examination Survey (HANES I). Evidence for an association with overweight, race, and physical demands of work. *Am J Epidemiol*. 1988;128:179-189.

28   Tepper S, Hochberg M. Factors associated with hip osteoarthritis: data from the first National Health and Nutrition Examination Survey (NHANES-I). *Am J Epidemiol*. 1993;137:1081-1088.

29   Bremner J, Lawrence J, Miall W. Degenerative joint disease in a Jamaican rural population. *Ann Rheum Dis*. 1968;27:326-332.

30   Solomon L, Beighton P, Lawrence J. Rheumatic disorders in the South African negro. Part II. Osteo-arthrosis. *S Afr Med J*. 1975;49:1737-1740.

31   Hoaglund F, Yau A, Wong W. Osteoarthritis of the hip and other joints in southern Chinese in Hong Kong. *J Bone Joint Surg Am*. 1973;55:545-557.

32   Nevitt M, Xu L, Zhang Y, et al. Very low prevalence of hip osteoarthritis among Chinese elderly in Beijing, China, compared with whites in the United States: the Beijing osteoarthritis study. *Arthritis Rheum*. 2002;46:1773-1779.

33   Zhang Y, Xu L, Nevitt M, et al. Lower prevalence of hand osteoarthritis among Chinese subjects in Beijing compared with white subjects in the United States: the Beijing osteoarthritis study. *Arthritis Rheum*. 2003;48:1034-1040.

34   Macgregor A, Antoniades L, Matson M, Andrew T, Spector T. The genetic contribution to radiographic hip osteoarthritis in women: results of a classic twin study. *Arthritis Rheum*. 2000;43:2410-2416.

35 Spector T, Cicuttini F, Baker J, Loughlin J, Hart D. Genetic influences on osteoarthritis in women: a twin study. *BMJ.* 1996;312:940-943.

36 Kaprio J, Kujala U, Peltonen L, Koskenvuo M. Genetic liability to osteoarthritis may be greater in women than men. *BMJ.* 1996;313:232.

37 Felson D, Couropmitree N, Chaisson C, et al. Evidence for a Mendelian gene in a segregation analysis of generalized radiographic osteoarthritis: the Framingham study. *Arthritis Rheum.* 1998;41:1064-1071.

38 Lanyon P, Muir K, Doherty S, Doherty M. Assessment of a genetic contribution to osteoarthritis of the hip: sibling study. *BMJ.* 2000;321:1179-1183.

39 Ingvarsson T, Stefansson S, Hallgrimsdottir I, et al. The inheritance of hip osteoarthritis in Iceland. *Arthritis Rheum.* 2000;43:2785-2792.

40 Jonsson H, Manolescu I, Stefansson S, et al. The inheritance of hand osteoarthritis in Iceland. *Arthritis Rheum.* 2003;48:391-395.

41 Loughlin J. Genetic epidemiology of primary osteoarthritis. *Curr Opin Rheumatol.* 2001;13:111-116.

42 Felson D, Zhang Y, Hannan M, et al. Risk factors for incident radiographic knee osteoarthritis in the elderly: the Framingham study. *Arthritis Rheum.* 1997;40:728-733.

43 Spector T, Hart D, Doyle D. Incidence and progression of osteoarthritis in women with unilateral knee disease in the general population: the effect of obesity. *Ann Rheum Dis.* 1994;53:565-568.

44 Gelber A, Hochberg M, Mead L, Wang N, Wigley F, Klag M. Body mass index in young men and the risk of subsequent knee and hip osteoarthritis. *Am J Med.* 1999;107:542-548.

45 Cooper C, Snow S, McAlindon T, et al. Risk factors for the incidence and progression of radiographic knee osteoarthritis. *Arthritis Rheum.* 2000;43:995-1000.

46 Schouten J, Van Den Ouweland FA, Valkenburg H. A 12 year follow up study in the general population on prognostic factors of cartilage loss in osteoarthritis of the knee. *Ann Rheum Dis.* 1992;51:932-937.

47 Harris W. Etiology of osteoarthritis of the hip. *Clin Orthop Relat Res.* 1986;213:20-33.

48 Andriacchi T. Dynamics of knee malalignment. *Orthop Clin North Am.* 1994;25:395-403.

49 Felson D, Nevitt M, Zhang Y, et al. High prevalence of lateral knee osteoarthritis in Beijing Chinese compared with Framingham caucasian subjects. *Arthritis Rheum.* 2002;46:1217-1222.

50 Sharma L, Song J, Felson D, Cahue S, Shamiyeh E, Dunlop D. The role of knee alignment in disease progression and functional decline in knee osteoarthritis. *JAMA.* 2001;286:188-195.

51 Bijlsma JWJ, Berenbaum F, Lafeber FPJG. Osteoarthritis: an update with relevance for clinical practice. *Lancet.* 2011;377:2115-2126.

52 Dam E, Loog M, Christiansen C, et al. Identification of progressors in osteoarthritis by combining biochemical and MRI-based markers. *Arthritis Res Ther.* 2009;11:R115.

53 Massardo L, Watt I, Cushnaghan J, Dieppe P. Osteoarthritis of the knee joint: an eight year prospective study. *Ann Rheum Dis.* 1989;48:893-897.

54 Spector TD, Dacre JE, Harris PA, Huskisson EC. Radiological progression of osteoarthritis: an 11 year follow up study of the knee. *Ann Rheum Dis.* 1992;51:1107-1110.

55 Thorstensson CA, Andersson ML, Jönsson H, Saxne T, Petersson IF. Natural course of knee osteoarthritis in middle-aged subjects with knee pain: 12-year follow-up using clinical and radiographic criteria. *Ann Rheum Dis.* 2009;68:1890-1893.

56 Hernborg JS, Nilsson BE. The natural course of untreated osteoarthritis of the knee. *Clin Orthop Relat Res.* 1977;123:130-137.

57 Lachance L, Sowers MF, Jamadar D, Hochberg M. The natural history of emergent osteoarthritis of the knee in women. *Osteoarthr Cartil.* 2002;10:849-854.

58 Felson DT, Zhang Y, Hannan MT, et al. The incidence and natural history of knee osteoarthritis in the elderly. The Framingham Osteoarthritis Study. *Arthritis Rheum.* 1995;38:1500-1505.

59 Danielsson L, Hernborg J. Morbidity and mortality of osteoarthritis of the knee (gonarthrosis) in Malmö, Sweden. *Clin Orthop Relat Res.* 1970;69:224-226.

60 Dougados M, Gueguen A, Nguyen M, et al. Longitudinal radiologic evaluation of osteoarthritis of the knee. *J Rheumatol.* 1992;19:378-384.

61 Spector TD, Hochberg MC. Methodological problems in the epidemiological study of osteoarthritis. *Ann Rheum Dis.* 1994;53:143-146.

62 Ledingham J, Regan M, Jones A, Doherty M. Factors affecting radiographic progression of knee osteoarthritis. *Ann Rheum Dis.* 1995;54:53-58.

63 McAlindon TE, Wilson PW, Aliabadi P, Weissman B, Felson DT. Level of physical activity and the risk of radiographic and symptomatic knee osteoarthritis in the elderly: the Framingham study. *Am J Med.* 1999;106:151-157.

64 Felson DT, Neogi T. Osteoarthritis: is it a disease of cartilage or of bone? *Arthritis Rheum.* 2004;50:341-344.

65 Dennison E, Cooper C. The natural history and prognosis of osteoarthritis. In: Brandt K, Doherty M, Lohmander M, eds. *Textbook of Osteoarthritis.* 2nd ed. Oxford: Oxford University Press; 2003:227-233.

66 Leyland KM, Hart DJ, Javaid MK, et al. The natural history of radiographic knee osteoarthritis: a fourteen-year population-based cohort study. *Arthritis Rheum.* 2012;64:2243-2251.

67 Soni A, Kiran A, Hart D, et al. Prevalence of reported knee pain over twelve years in a community-based cohort. *Arthritis Rheum.* 2012;64:1145-1152.

68 Bayliss E, Ellis J, Steiner J. Barriers to self-management and quality-of-life outcomes in seniors with multimorbidities. *Ann Fam Med.* 2007;5:395-402.

69 Datamonitor. Stakeholder Insight: Osteoarthritis. Drug development lags behind rising osteoarthritis population. Datamonitor Europe: London, UK; December 2009.

Chapter 3
Pathophysiology of osteoarthritis

Francois Rannou

Anatomy of normal joints

Human movement is made possible by synovial fluid, or freely moving, and cartilaginous, or fixed, joints [1]. The synovial joint is a functional connective tissue unit that allows two opposed limb bones to move freely in relation to each other. The bone–cartilage–synovial fluid–cartilage–bone assembly can be regarded as a continuum, with the load-bearing structures organised differently depending on site and function, resulting in a specialised joint structure [1].

There are five basic types of structures in the knee (Figures 3.1 and 3.2, see page 36) [2–5]:

- ligaments, which are passive elastic structures that can be loaded in tension only;
- musculotendinous units, which are active elastic structures that act only under tension;
- cartilage and subchondral bone, which accommodate the compressive loads of the joint;
- menisci, which are crescentic fibrocartilaginous pads that attach to the intercondylar area and periphery of the tibial plateau; and
- the bursae.

Anterior and lateral view of the normal knee anatomy

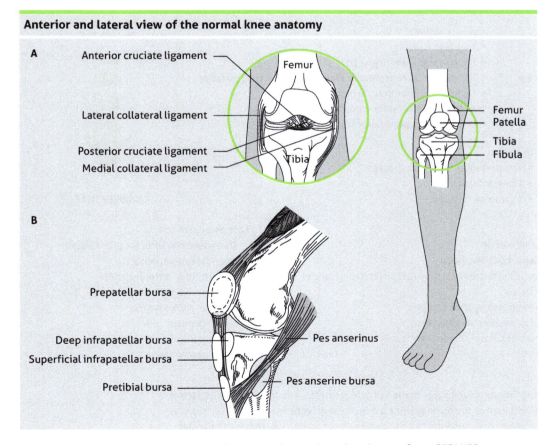

Figure 3.1 Anterior and lateral view of the normal knee anatomy.
A, image showing the basic structure of the knee. Ligaments can be divided into intra-articular and extracapsular.
B, The major bursae around the knee. Adapted with permission from Niitsu [5].

This publication has been made possible through an educational grant from SERVIER.

N. Arden et al., *Atlas of Osteoarthritis*, DOI 10.1007/978-1-910315-16-3_3,
© Springer Healthcare 2014

Plain radiograph of the normal right knee

Femur

Patella

Tibia

Fibula

Figure 3.2 Plain radiograph of the normal right knee. This radiograph clearly shows the femur, tibia and fibula. The patella can be seen as faint circular outline overlapping the femur, centred at the widest part of the femur. Image from Abdul-Jabar et al [4].

Pathophysiology

Osteoarthritis is considered an organ disease that involves the whole joint structure. A gradual loss of articular cartilage in synovial joints is combined with subchondral bone sclerosis, osteophytes at the joint margins and mild, chronic nonspecific synovial inflammation [6,7]. A hypothetical model of the development of osteoarthritis is shown in Figure 3.3 [6].

Hypothetical model for initiation and perpetuation of osteoarthritis

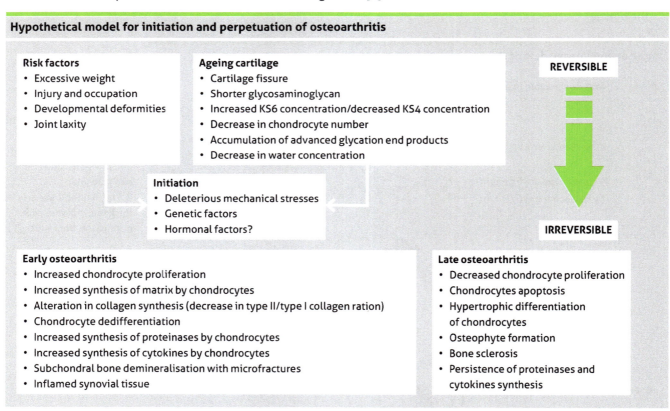

Risk factors
- Excessive weight
- Injury and occupation
- Developmental deformities
- Joint laxity

Ageing cartilage
- Cartilage fissure
- Shorter glycosaminoglycan
- Increased KS6 concentration/decreased KS4 concentration
- Decrease in chondrocyte number
- Accumulation of advanced glycation end products
- Decrease in water concentration

Initiation
- Deleterious mechanical stresses
- Genetic factors
- Hormonal factors?

REVERSIBLE

IRREVERSIBLE

Early osteoarthritis
- Increased chondrocyte proliferation
- Increased synthesis of matrix by chondrocytes
- Alteration in collagen synthesis (decrease in type II/type I collagen ration)
- Chondrocyte dedifferentiation
- Increased synthesis of proteinases by chondrocytes
- Increased synthesis of cytokines by chondrocytes
- Subchondral bone demineralisation with microfractures
- Inflamed synovial tissue

Late osteoarthritis
- Decreased chondrocyte proliferation
- Chondrocytes apoptosis
- Hypertrophic differentiation of chondrocytes
- Osteophyte formation
- Bone sclerosis
- Persistence of proteinases and cytokines synthesis

Figure 3.3 Hypothetical model for initiation and perpetuation of osteoarthritis. Accumulation of risk factors on ageing cartilage triggers the initiation of the osteoarthritic process. For didactic reasons, two phases are described, early osteoarthritis and late osteoarthritis, but the passage from one to the other is progressive and generally lasts many years. KS, keratan sulphate. Reproduced with permission from Berenbaum [6].

Osteoarthritis is often thought of as a degenerative condition, but does not arise just because of gradual wear and tear. Instead, it should be looked at as an abnormal remodelling of the joint tissues, articular cartilage and bone, which is driven by many inflammatory mediators [8].

The development of osteoarthritis is usually related to one of two fundamental mechanisms connected to the adverse effects of 'abnormal' loading on 'normal' cartilage or 'normal' loading on 'abnormal' cartilage. Ageing may be the main contributing factor to 'abnormal' articular cartilage, but genetic factors that influence the structure and composition of the cartilage matrix and which cause disruption of chondrocyte differentiation and function can also contribute to abnormal biomechanics [9]. Normal loading on abnormal cartilage, or structural instability due to repetitive joint traumatism, is a main cause of osteoarthritis in younger people [10].

Joint structural changes

The radiographic features of osteoarthritis include (Figure 3.4) [11]:

- narrowing of the joint space;
- cysts in the subchondral bone;
- bone condensation in the contact area; and
- osteophytosis in the non-contact area.

Radiographic manifestations of osteoarthritis

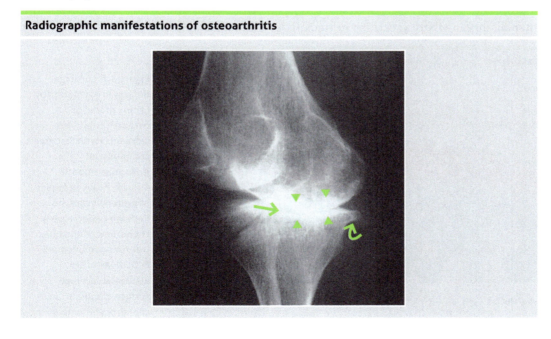

Figure 3.4 Radiographic manifestations of osteoarthritis. This oblique radiograph of the right knee shows marked narrowing of the medial femorotibial compartment (open arrow) with subchondral condensation (arrowheads) and a marginal osteophyte at the posterior tibial edge (curved arrow). Reproduced with permission from Bahk [11].

The most commonly affected sites are the hand, knee and hip [12]. Another important site is the spine, with degenerative changes often seen in the intervertebral disc of the lower lumbar and lumbrosacral vertebrae and the apophyseal and costovertebral joints. Figure 3.5 shows the radiographical changes associated with discovertebral osteoarthritis [11] (see page 38).

Cartilage degradation

Under normal conditions, the physiologic homeostasis of the articular cartilage is driven by chondrocytes, which produce the structural matrix containing collagens (primarily collagen

Discovertebral osteoarthritis of the spine

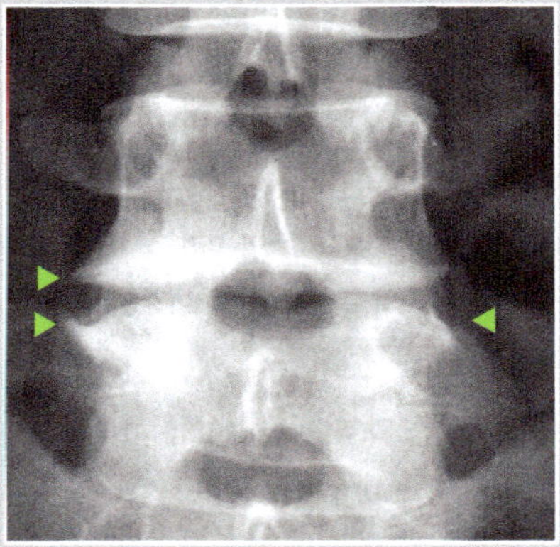

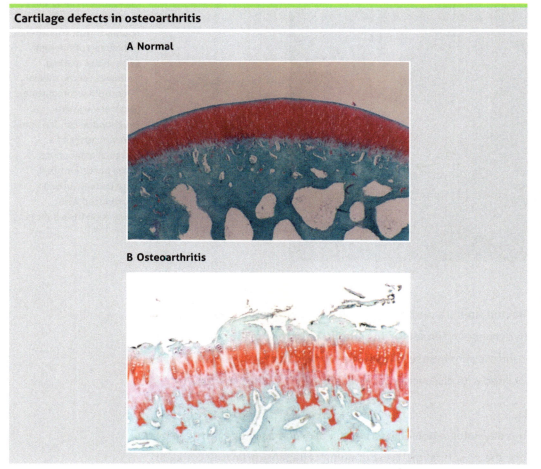

Figure 3.5 Discovertebral osteoarthritis of the spine. Anteroposterior radiograph of the lower lumbar spine shows endplate-based sclerosis in the L4 lower and L5 upper end-plates with narrowing of the disc space between them (arrow). Small claw-like spurs (arrowheads) are seen at the right lateral edges. Reproduced with permission from Bahk [11].

type II), and proteoglycans [6,13]. Despite the involvement of multiple joint tissues, osteoarthritis has long been mainly characterised by a breakdown of the repair process of damaged cartilage as a result of biochemical and biomechanical changes in the joint [12]. The changes in cartilage structure as a result of osteoarthritis are shown in Figure 3.6 [13].

In osteoarthritis, the chondrocytes within the joint fail to synthesise a resistant and elastic matrix and therefore cannot maintain the balance between synthesis and degradation of the extracellular matrix [6]. Inflammatory mediators such as interleukin (IL)-1 and mechanical

Cartilage defects in osteoarthritis

A Normal

B Osteoarthritis

Figure 3.6 Cartilage defects in osteoarthritis. Lapine model of osteoarthritis using safranin O with fast green counterstain.
A, Normal: smooth surface, heavy red stain of proteoglycans, no increase or decrease in chondrocytes and one well-defined tidemark.
B, Osteoarthritis: disrupted cartilage surface, proliferation of chondrocytes with many pyknotic chondrocytes (indicating cell death), sparse red stain of proteoglycans that is only present around chondrocytes, and duplicated tidemark invaded by blood vessels. Reproduced with permission from Altman [13].

stress then drive chondrocytes to produce less functional collagen (collagen type I), smaller and less space-occupying proteoglycans, more degradative enzymes and multiple mediators of inflammation, including nitric oxide and additional IL-1 [13]. This causes a vicious cycle in which breakdown exceeds synthesis of the extracellular matrix [12], leading to loss of articular cartilage (Figure 3.7) [14]. As articular cartilage is aneural, these changes do not result in clinical signs unless innervated tissues become involved [12].

Loss of articular cartilage in osteoarthritis

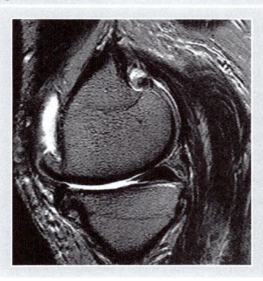

Figure 3.7 Loss of articular cartilage in osteoarthritis. In this magnetic resonance image of a knee with advanced osteoarthritis, the triangular posterior horn of the medial meniscus is in contact with the cortical margin of the subchondral bone, which appears black. This suggests that little or no articular cartilage remains on the posterior aspect of the femoral condyle. Reproduced with permission from Myers [14].

Some of the molecular changes seen in cartilage from osteoarthritic joints may be the result of the ageing process itself. While ageing does cause the wear and tear that precipitates osteoarthritis, there are also theories that suggest that there are programmed changes in chondrocytes that take years to manifest (eg, apoptosis). These changes may leave cartilage more vulnerable to degeneration even in the absence of undue joint stress [10].

The role of subchondral bone changes in osteoarthritis

The role of subchondral bone is currently believed to be of particular importance in the pathogenesis of osteoarthritis. Subchondral bone performs shock-absorbing and support duties in normal joints and supplies nutrients to cartilage [15]. It lies immediately beneath the calcified cartilage and is a plate of cortical bone that is physiologically and mechanically similar to cortical bone in other skeletal locations but is not as stiff as diaphyseal cortical bone. Distal to this cortical bone plate is subchondral cancellous bone that is more porous and metabolically active and has a lower density, volume and stiffness. The term 'subchondral bone' refers to both these cortical and cancellous parts [16].

Both early-stage increased bone remodelling and subchondral bone loss, and late-stage slow remodelling and subchondral sclerosis (a long-recognised hallmark of osteoarthritis) are important components of the pathogenetic process that leads to osteoarthritis [12,16]. However, it remains unclear as to whether changes in the subchondral bone occur before cartilage degradation or result from it. Data from various animal studies demonstrate that microstructural subchondral bone alterations may occur before, during or after cartilage damage [16].

41

Subchondral bone in different stages of osteoarthritis

In early osteoarthritis, an increased rate of bone remodelling is observed, associated with a transient loss of bone, increased porosity in the subchondral region and reduced density, leading to a decrease in the subchondral plate thickness (Figure 3.8) [16]. In canine models, this thinning in subchondral bone has been associated with increased cartilage destruction and reduced synthesis of glycosaminoglycans [17].

The causes of increased bone remodelling in early osteoarthritis are unknown, but several different mechanisms are suspected:

- Cellular signalling: elevated levels of mediators of inflammation (eg, IL-1 and IL-6) that are both stimulators and products of bone remodelling have been detected in deteriorating cartilage [16]. There is evidence to suggest that microcracks in the subchondral plate caused by normal joint loading can stimulate osteocytes to produce receptor activator of nuclear factor κ-B ligand (RANKL) and downregulate osteoprotegerin, thus inducing bone resorption [16]. RANKL and its isoforms are differentially expressed in subchondral bone osteoblasts taken from patients with osteoarthritis [18].

- Vascular invasion: subchondral bone is a richly vascularised tissue, and microvascular changes are a well described part of the early pathology of osteoarthritis [19]. Increased bone remodelling is associated with vascular invasion and this increased vascularity, if unchecked, can lead to vessels invading the deep layers of articular cartilage (which is usually avascular). This proangiogenic milieu can induce chondrocytes to synthesise catabolic enzymes such as matrix metalloproteinases (MMPs), resulting in cartilage degeneration [16]. Secondary to this process, vascular invasion of the cartilage may also diminish the mechanical integrity of the cartilage matrix. Taken together, these changes can create a positive feedback loop as bone remodelling continues to occur to help the joint adapt to the altered loads [16].

    - The complexity of osteoarthritis vascular abnormalities is compounded by the observation that atheromatous vascular disease is linked to osteoarthritis. Accordingly, it has been hypothesised that vascular disease in subchondral bone may accelerate the disease process, either by altering cartilage nutrition or through direct ischaemic effects on bone [19].

Stages of progressive joint and subchondral bone degradation in osteoarthritis

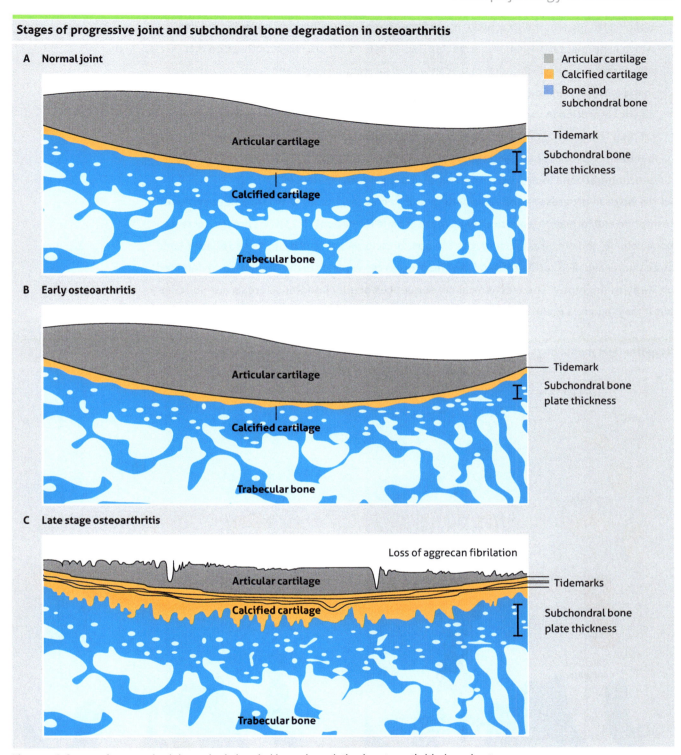

Figure 3.8 Stages of progressive joint and subchondral bone degradation in osteoarthritis. In early-stage osteoarthritis, the subchondral plate becomes thinner as a consequence of an increased remodelling rate. At the same time, cancellous bone is lost as the trabecular plates become thinner and more rod-like. In late-stage disease, the subchondral plate thickens, but the subchondral cancellous bone remains osteopaenic. The calcified cartilage begins to advance into the articular cartilage, leaving a footprint of multiple tidemarks as the mineralisation front advances. This creates an even thicker mineralised plate, and reduces the thickness of the non-mineralised articular cartilage, which cannot replace itself. This is accompanied by surface fibrillation and a loss of aggrecan, beginning superficially in the articular cartilage. The collective result of these changes is subchondral sclerosis (that includes both the subchondral plate and calcified cartilage) and thinner, more fibrillated articular cartilage. Image from Burr & Gallant [16]. © 2012, reproduced with permission from Nature Publishing Group.

- Bone–cartilage crosstalk: cartilage is separated from the subchondral bone by a tidemark, which in normal cartilage is impermeable [20]. In osteoarthritis, it is hypothesised that microcracks in the subchondral plate can lead to interactions between bone and cartilage in the early phase of disease. These microcracks may be further exacerbated by the osteoclastic resorption in the subchondral region, which leads to increased plate perforation [16,21]. This theory is substantiated by in vitro studies showing that there is crosstalk between cells of the bone and chondrocytes [16]. A hypothetical model of cartilage and subchondral bone interaction in osteoarthritis is given in Figure 3.9 [22].

As the disease progresses, the remodelling rate decreases, but an imbalance between bone resorption and formation leads to a net increase in bone formation [16,23]. This process increases bone volume, and can be associated with an apparent sclerosis caused by increased bone volume and a thicker calcified cartilage layer [16]. This process corresponds to the condensation detected on X-ray radiography. The mechanical consequences of subchondral sclerosis are not clear but it may lead to a greater bone volume, with lower mineralisation, in joints of patients with

Hypothetical model of cartilage and subchondral bone interaction in osteoarthritis

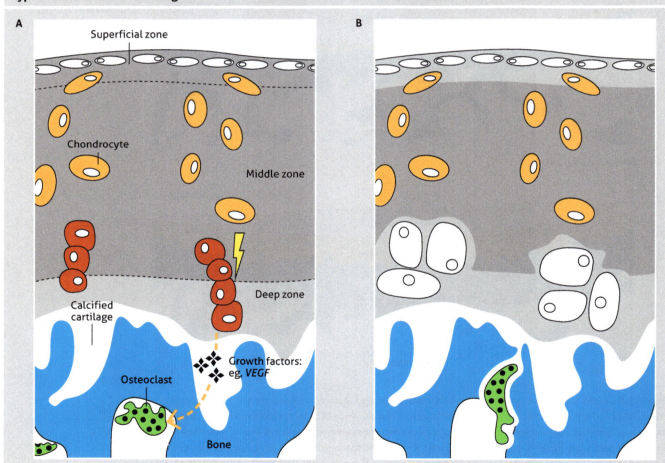

osteoarthritis compared with disease-free joints, leading to diminished mechanical stiffness of the bone and, consequently, deterioration of cartilage [16].

During this stage, osteophytes may develop at the joint margins [13]. Osteophytes are outgrowths of osseous tissue that are covered with cartilage [24]. Types of osteophytes include traction spurs at the attachment of the ligament and tendon to bone, inflammatory spurs in the vertebral body and osteochondrophytes, which form from metaplasia of the synovium into cartilage. Their role in osteoarthritis is unclear; they could cause pain in spinal osteoarthritis but may be helpful in osteoarthritis of the lower limbs because they stabilise the joint [25].

Synovial inflammation in osteoarthritis

The synovial membrane plays a key role in normal joint function, as it nourishes chondrocytes through the synovial fluid and joint space and eliminates metabolites and matrix degradation products [26]. Hyaluronic acid and lubricin produced in the synovial lining cells help protect and maintain articular cartilage [27].

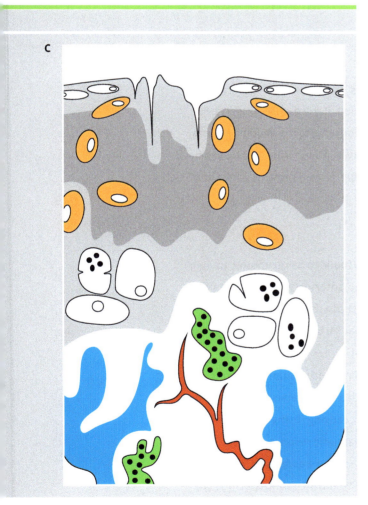

Figure 3.9 Hypothetical model of cartilage and subchondral bone interaction in osteoarthritis.
A, Healthy chondrocytes under pathological conditions (eg, due to instability of the joint or severe increased mobilisation) start to become hypertrophic and produce growth factors that diffuse towards the underlying bone marrow and stimulate osteoclastogenesis.
B, Persisting strain. Chondrocytes become more hypertrophic and produce less sulphated-glycosaminoglycans (sGAG) to sustain the cartilage. Osteoclasts start to tunnel through the subchondral bone inducing changes to the biomechanical properties of the tissue.
C, Progressive phase of osteoarthritis. The tidemark between cartilage and bone shifts upwards, reducing cartilage thickness. The remaining cartilage is strongly depleted of sGAG and becomes structurally deprived. Osteoclast activity extends into the calcified cartilage, up to the border with the deep zone of the cartilage. Via the pores there is vascular ingrowth into the cartilage. Later on, osteoblasts will infiltrate and start to deposit bone that results in end-stage sclerosis. Image from Weinans et al [22]. © 2012, reproduced with permission from Elsevier.

Involvement of the synovium in osteoarthritis pathophysiology

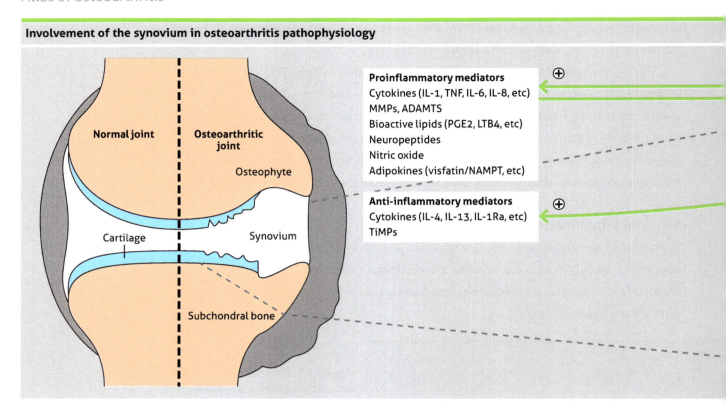

The inflammation of the synovium that occurs in osteoarthritis is responsible for several clinical symptoms, including pain, and reflects the structural progression of the disorder [26,27]. Furthermore, synovitis is a major factor in osteoarthritis pathophysiology due to the action of several soluble mediators (Figure 3.10). Interestingly, the relationship between synovitis, as assessed by arthroscopy, and the degree of functional impairment or pain experienced remains a matter of debate [26].

Ligament changes and misalignment

About one-quarter of patients with knee osteoarthritis have been found to have ruptures to their anterior cruciate ligament (ACL), which normally functions as an anterior/posterior stabiliser [28,29]. A detailed study of the effect of ageing and osteoarthritis on the ACL found moderate or severe degeneration of the ACL in knees that had only minimal cartilage deterioration. The likelihood of advanced ACL degeneration increased with age [29].

Patients with established knee osteoarthritis may also have varus alignment, causing medial tibiofemoral osteoarthritis, and/or valgus alignment, which leads to lateral osteoarthritis progression [30]. Both of these conditions affect load distribution, causing further knee damage. In one trial of 256 patients with knee osteoarthritis who had no magnetic resonance image (MRI) evidence of tibiofemoral cartilage damage, varus alignment at baseline was associated with an increased risk of incident medial tibiofemoral cartilage damage over a 30-month period [30].

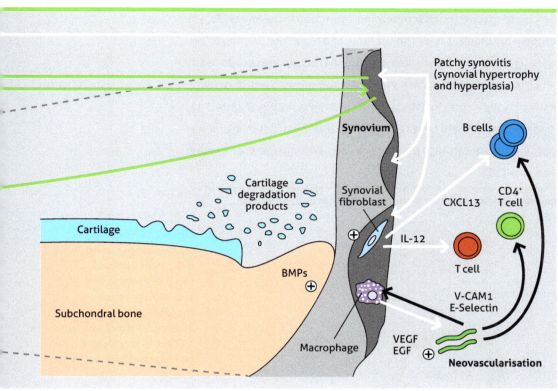

Figure 3.10 Involvement of the synovium in osteoarthritis pathophysiology. Products of cartilage breakdown that are released into the synovial fluid are phagocytosed by synovial cells, amplifying synovial inflammation. In turn, activated synovial cells produce catabolic and pro-inflammatory mediators, leading to excess production of the proteolytic enzymes responsible for cartilage breakdown. This inflammatory response is amplified by activated synovial T cells, B cells and infiltrating macrophages; to counteract it, the synovium and cartilage produce anti-inflammatory cytokines. The inflamed synovium also contributes to the formation of osteophytes via BMPs. ADAMTS, a disintegrin and metalloproteinase with thrombospondin motifs; BMP, bone morphogenetic protein; CCL2, CC-chemokine ligand 2; CXCL13, CXC-chemokine ligand 13; EGF, endothelial growth factor; GM-CSF, granulocyte-macrophage colony-stimulating factor; IL, interleukin; IL-1Ra, IL-1 receptor antagonist; LIF, leukaemia inhibitory factor; LTB4, leukotriene B4; MMP, matrix metalloproteinase; NAMPT, nicotinamide phosphoribosyl transferase (also called visfatin); NGF, nerve growth factor; PGE2, prostaglandin E2; TIMP, tissue inhibitor of metalloproteinase; TNF, tumour necrosis factor; VCAM-1, vascular cell adhesion molecule 1; VEGF, vascular endothelial growth factor. Image from Sellam & Berenbaum [26]. © 2010, reproduced with permission from Nature Publishing Group.

Risk factors for osteoarthritis

Many risk factors are associated with the development and progression of osteoarthritis (Table 3.1) [12]. Age, female gender, participation in intense sports activities and high body mass index (obesity) are among the many factors linked to both development and progression [12,31]. Sex hormones may play a role in the accelerated incidence rate of osteoarthritis in postmenopausal women [31].

Selected risk factors for the occurrence and progression of osteoarthritis in knee, hip and hand

	Knee	Hip	Hand
Occurrence	Age, sex, physical activity, body-mass index (including obesity), intense sport activities, quadriceps strength, bone density, previous injury, hormone replacement therapy (protective), vitamin D, smoking (protective or deleterious), malalignment (including varus and valgus), genetics	Age, sex, physical activity, body-mass index (including obesity), previous injury, intense sport activities, genetics (including congenital deformities)	Age, grip strength, occupation, intense sport activities, genetics
Progression	Age, body-mass index (including obesity), vitamin D, hormone replacement therapy (protective), malalignment (including varus and valgus), chronic joint effusion, synovitis, intense sport activities, subchondral bone oedema on magnetic resonance imaging	Age, symptomatic activity, sex, intense sport activities	Unknown

Table 3.1 Selected risk factors for the occurrence and progression of osteoarthritis in knee, hip and hand. The risk factors involved in the occurrence and progression of osteoarthritis differ depending on the joint(s) involved. Reproduced with permission from Bijlsma et al [12].

Obesity is a recognised cause of osteoarthritis progression, especially in the knees [31,32]. The extra weight places additional mechanical stress on the knee and hip joints, leading to cartilage breakdown and damaged ligaments [31]. Data also indicate that adipokines produced by fat cells (eg, leptin, restin), which are involved in glucose and lipid metabolism as well as modulation of inflammatory responses, may play a role in osteoarthritis pathophysiology (Figure 3.11) [32]. People who are obese and then lose weight have less cartilage thickness loss in the medial femoral compartment and improved medial cartilage proteoglycan content, regardless of whether they have osteoarthritis at baseline [33].

Schematic representation network linking white adipose tissue dysfunction, bone and cartilage tissues

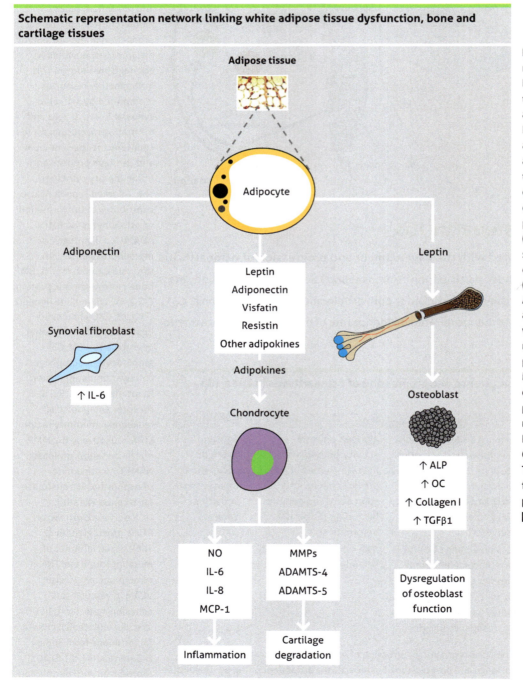

Figure 3.11 Schematic representation network linking white adipose tissue dysfunction, bone and cartilage tissues. Dysfunctional fat produces an excess of proinflammatory adipokines that are able to interact with bone cells, synovial cells and chondrocytes by inducing proinflammatory mediators (cytokines, reactive oxygen species, NO) and cartilage degradative factors (MMPs and ADAMTSs). ADAMTS, a disintegrin and metalloproteinase with thrombospondin motifs; ALP, alkaline phosphatase; IL, interleukin; MCP, monocyte chemoattractant protein; MMPs, matrix metalloproteinases; NO, nitric oxide; OC, osteocalcin; TGF, transforming growth factor. Reproduced with permission from Conde et al [32].

Molecular mechanisms of osteoarthritis development

While ageing *per se* is not viewed as the initiating factor for the development of osteoarthritis, age-related changes within the chondrocyte, such as cellular senescence and a reduced responsiveness to growth factors, as well as external factors such as the accumulation of advanced glycation end products and oxidative stress, may combine to disrupt cartilage homeostasis (Table 3.2) [34–53]. These changes make the cartilage matrix more vulnerable to damage and lead to the onset of osteoarthritis (Figure 3.12; see page 48) [34].

Molecular events in articular chondrocytes associated with ageing

Phenotype of chondrocyte ageing	Molecular events
Altered gene expression related to senescence	• ↑ GADD45β and C/EBPβ → ↑ p21 transcription [35] • ↓ SIRT1→↑ p53, ↑ p21 [36] • ↑ Caveolin 1→↑ p53, ↑ p21 [37] • ↑ β-Galactosidase [38]
DNA and telomere dysfunction	• ↓ TRF → telomere shortening [36] • ↓ XRCC5→↑ DNA damage [36] • Mitochondrial DNA degradation [38]
Altered protein secretion	• ↑ Pro-inflammatory cytokines (ie, IL-1β, TNF-α) and pro-inflammatory mediators (PGE2, NO) [39] • ↑ MMPs (−1, −3, −13) and ADAMTS (−4, −5) [40,41]
Oxidative damage	• ↑ ROS production [42,43] • ↓ Antioxidant enzyme activity [44] • Mitochondrial dysfunction [45]
↓ Growth factor response	• Impaired responsiveness to IGF-1 [46,47], OP-1/BMP-7 [48], TGF-β [49,50]
Cell death	• ↓ IGF-1 and OP-1 → reduced cellularity [51] • ↓ CK2→apoptosis [52] • ↓ HMGB2→apoptosis [53]

Table 3.2 Molecular events in articular chondrocytes associated with ageing. During the ageing process, chondrocytes exhibit features consistent with a senescent phenotype. These changes impair the ability of chondrocytes to maintain the surrounding extracellular matrix. ADAMTS, a disintegrin and metalloproteinase with thrombospondin motifs; BMP-7, bone morphogenic protein-7; C/EBPβ, CCAAT/enhancer binding protein β; GADD45β, growth arrest and DNA damage-inducible 45β; HMGB2, high-mobility group box protein 2, insulin-like growth factor-1; IL-1β, interleukin-1β; MMPs, matrix metalloproteinases; NO, nitric oxide; OP-1, osteogenic protein-1; PGE2, prostaglandin E2; ROS, reactive oxygen species; SIRT1, sirtuin 1; TGF-β, transforming growth factor-β; TNF-α, tumour necrosis factor-α; TRF, telomeric repeat binding factor; XRCC5, X-ray repair complementing defective repair in Chinese hamster cells 5. Reproduced with permission from Leong & Sun [34].

A potential model for osteoarthritis is one where it is represented as a chronic wound that triggers an innate immune response [54]. Recent data suggest that the matrix fragments and products released during cellular stress can activate the innate immune response via toll-like receptors. The ensuing cellular response culminates in the activation of specific transcription factors, most prominently nuclear factor κ-B, leading to production of multiple potent proinflammatory mediators that can cause local tissue damage [27].

Chondrocyte ageing and cartilage destruction

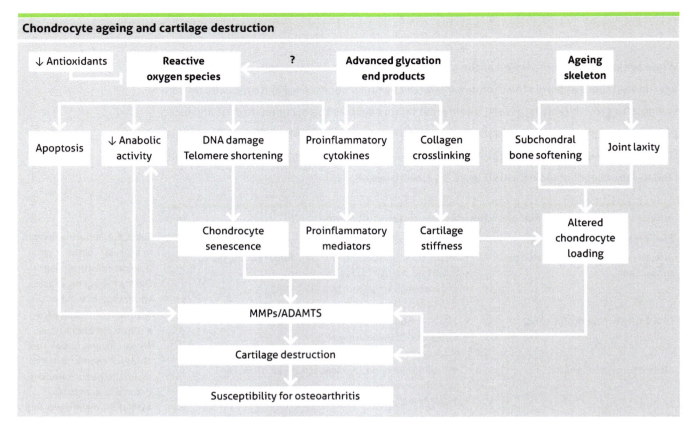

Figure 3.12 Chondrocyte ageing and cartilage destruction. Age-related changes in the cartilage extracellular matrix and surrounding joint tissues initiate a cascade of events within the articular chondrocyte that lead to cartilage destruction and potential development of osteoarth ritis. ADAMTS, a disintegrin and metalloproteinase with thrombospondin motifs; MMPs, matrix metalloproteinases. Reproduced with permission from Leong & Sun [34].

Cytokines (primarily interleukins and tumour necrosis factor-α), proteinases (primarily MMPs), lipid mediators and reactive oxygen species all stimulate chondrocytes to release cartilage-degrading enzymes [6,55]. An analysis of osteoblasts derived from osteophytes demonstrates that IL-6, IL-8 and MMP-13 levels are greatly increased in patients with osteoarthritis (Figure 3.13) [24]. Applying nonphysical mechanical stress loads to osteoblasts also increases the gene expression of IL-6 and IL-8 in a stress magnitude-dependent manner, further demonstrating the significance of inflammatory factors in osteophytes. Moreover, IL-6 directly induces MMP-13 expression and production in osteoarthritis osteoblasts from osteophytes and subchondral bone osteoblasts without osteoarthritis [24]. The increased expression of IL-8 and MMP-13 may promote cartilage degeneration via chondrocyte hypertrophy [24].

Growth factors involved in the synthesis of the physiological matrix, such as insulin-like growth factor-1, bone morphogenic proteins, platelet-derived growth factor and transforming growth factor-β can inhibit the effects of proinflammatory cytokines and help to repair the cartilage damage associated with osteoarthritis [6,55]. They stimulate chondrocyte anabolic activity and proteoglycan synthesis and may also inhibit catabolic activity [55].

Currently, there is no reliable biomarker that can be considered a valid tool for the diagnosis and prognosis of osteoarthritis in routine clinical practice. However, fibulin-3 peptides and

Concentrations of IL-6, IL-8 and MMP-13 in culture supernatant of osteoblasts isolated from osteophytes of patients with osteoarthritis

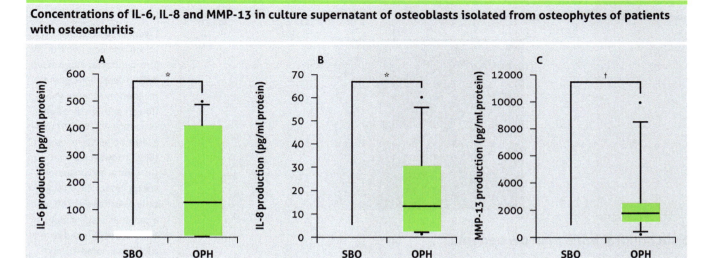

Figure 3.13 Concentrations of IL-6, IL-8 and MMP-13 in culture supernatant of osteoblasts isolated from osteophytes of patients with osteoarthritis. IL-6 (**A**), IL-8 (**B**) and MMP-13 (**C**) levels in osteoarthritis osteoblasts (OPH) were significantly higher than those of osteoblasts from subchondral bone without osteoarthritis (SBO; $P<0.05$, <0.05 and <0.01, respectively). The IL-8 and MMP-13 levels in the cell culture supernatant of osteoblasts from subchondral bone without osteoarthritis were below the limits of detection. *$P<0.05$, †$P<0.01$ (SBO, n=3; OPH, n=7). IL, Interleukin; MMPs, matrix metalloproteinases. Data from Sakao et al [24]. © 2009, reproduced with permission from The Japanese Society for Bone and Mineral Research and Springer.

follistatin-like protein-1 (FSTL1), both extracellular proteins, have potential as osteoarthritis bio-markers [56]. Fibulin 3 is widely distributed in various tissue types and blood vessels of different sizes and is capable of inhibiting vessel development and angiogenesis. Furthermore, it is also elevated in osteoarthritis cartilage. In a recent study, Henrotin et al found greater levels of two fibulin 3 fragments (Fib3-1 and Fib3-2) in the urine and serum of patients with osteoarthritis than in controls. The increased levels of Fib3-1 were associated with ageing and hormonal status, but Fib3-2 levels were not modified by gender, age or menopause [57]. FSTL1 is expressed in human tissues and is induced by ischaemic stress and proinflammatory mediators [58]. It is thought to play a role in arthritis pathogenesis and has been found to be a biomarker for rheumatoid arthritis and other autoimmune diseases, as serum FSTL1 levels correlate with inflammatory status [58,59]. Serum FSTL1 levels have been found to be much higher in patients with osteoarthritis than in healthy controls, and in women were correlated with disease grade and joint space widening [58].

Osteoarthritis pain

The best radiological predictor of knee pain is the presence of osteophytes [60,61], with the strongest association observed in the skyline view compared with the lateral or anteroposterior views [61]. The presence of osteophytes on any view is a better predictor of knee pain than joint space width [60,61]. It has been suggested that the induction of synovitis due to greater expression of IL-6 and IL-8 may also be a factor in the pain associated with osteoarthritis [24].

Bone marrow lesion in knee osteoarthritis

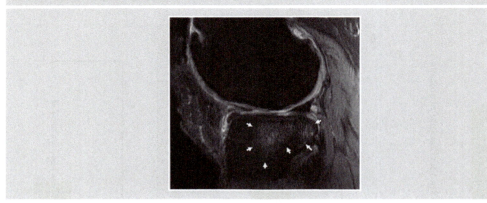

Figure 3.14 Bone marrow lesion in knee osteoarthritis. This sagittal fat-suppressed proton density-weighted magnetic resonance image (long repetition time/long echo time = 3500/20) shows a large bone marrow lesion (BML; arrows) involving the central and posterior subregions of the lateral tibia. Subchondral BMLs are a common imaging feature of osteoarthritis and several trials have noted a cross-sectional positive association between BMLs, cartilage damage and ligament damage. Importantly, BMLs in the knee have also been associated with pain. Image from Xu et al [63]. © 2012, reproduced with permission from Elsevier.

Subchondral bone marrow oedema

Bone contains pain fibres, and subchondral bone marrow oedema-like lesions (BMLs) have been frequently noted in osteoarthritis (Figure 3.14) [62,63]. Several trials have noted a cross-sectional positive association between BMLs, cartilage damage and ligament damage [63].

In a pivotal study involving 351 patients with osteoarthritis and knee pain and 50 patients with osteoarthritis but no knee pain, 78% of patients with knee pain had MRI evidence of bone marrow lesions, compared with only 30% of patients without knee pain ($P<0.001$) [62]. These results show that BMLs in the knee are associated with pain, the most important symptom of osteoarthritis. In addition, bone marrow lesions are correlated with the severity of radiographic disease. In this study, the prevalence of BMLs ranged from 48% in knees with Kellgren and Lawrence (KL) grades of 0 to 100% in knees with KL grades of 4 [62].

References

1   Gardner DL. Problems and paradigms in joint pathology. *J Anat.* 1994;184:465-476.
2   McLeod WD, Hunter S. Biomechanical analysis of the knee: primary functions as elucidated by anatomy. *Phys Ther.* 1980;60:1561-1564.
3   Kishner S, Courseault J, Authement A. Knee joint anatomy. Available at: http://emedicine.medscape.com/article/1898986-overview. Last accessed December 7, 2012.
4   Abdul-Jabar HB, Walsh U, Rashid A, Rajkumar S. Primary meningococcal osteoarthritis of the knee—case report and review of the literature. *Eur Orthop Traumatol.* 2011;2:149-152.
5   Niitsu M. Cystic and cyst-like lesions of the knee. In: Niitsu M, ed. *Magnetic Resonance Imaging of the Knee.* Springer-Verlag Berlin Heidelberg; 2013: 181-198.
6   Berenbaum F. Osteoarthritis. B. Pathology and pathogenesis. In: Klippel JH, Stone JH, Crofford LJ, White PH, eds. *Primer on the Rheumatic Diseases.* New York, NY: Springer Science+Business Media, LLC; 2008:229-234.
7   Symmons D, Mathers C, Pfleger B. Global burden of osteoarthritis in the year 2000. World Health Organization Web site. Available at: www.who.int/healthinfo/statistics/bod_osteoarthritis.pdf. Accessed December 7, 2012.
8   Loeser RF, Goldring SR, Scanzello CR, Goldring MB. Osteoarthritis: a disease of the joint as an organ. *Arthritis Rheum.* 2012;64:1697-1707.
9   Goldring MB, Goldring SR. Osteoarthritis. *J Cell Physiol.* 2007;213:626-634.
10 Horton WE Jr, Bennion P, Yang L. Cellular, molecular, and matrix changes in cartilage during aging and osteoarthritis. *J Musculoskelet Neuronal Interact.* 2006;6:379-381.
11 Bahk Y-W. Degenerative joint diseases. In: Bahk Y-W, ed. *Combined Scintigraphic and Radiographic Diagnosis of Bone and Joint Diseases, Including Gamma Correction Interpretation.* 4th ed. Berlin, Germany: Springer-Verlag Berlin Heidelberg; 2013:141-183.

12 Bijlsma JWJ, Berenbaum F, Lafeber FPJG. Osteoarthritis: an update with relevance for clinical practice. *Lancet*. 2011;377:2115-2126.

13 Altman RD. Osteoarthritis in the elderly population. In: Nakasato Y, Yung RL, eds. *Geriatric Rheumatology. A Comprehensive Approach*. New York, NY: Springer Science+Business Media, LLC; 2011:187-196.

14 Myers SL. Osteoarthritis and crystal-associated synovitis. In: Hunder GG, ed. *Atlas of Rheumatology*, 4th ed. Philadelphia, PA: Current Medicine LLC; 2005:54-81.

15 Castañeda S, Roman-Blas JA, Largo R, Herrero-Beaumont G. Subchondral bone as a key target for osteoarthritis treatment. *Biochem Pharmacol*. 2012;83:315-323.

16 Burr DB, Gallant MA. Bone remodelling in osteoarthritis. *Nat Rev Rheumatol*. 2012;8:665-673.

17 Sniekers YH, Intema F, Lafeber FPJG, et al. A role for subchondral bone changes in the process of osteoarthritis; a micro-CT study of two canine models. *BMC Musculoskelet Disord*. 2008;9:20.

18 Tat SK, Pelletier J-P, Lajeunesse D, Fahmi H, Duval N, Martel-Pelletier J. Differential modulation of RANKL isoforms by human osteoarthritic subchondral bone osteoblasts: influence of osteotropic factors. *Bone*. 2008;43:284-291.

19 Conaghan PG, Vanharanta H, Dieppe PA. Is progressive osteoarthritis an atheromatous vascular disease? *Ann Rheum Dis*. 2005;64:1539-1541.

20 Walsh D. Neurogenic factors in the etiopathogenesis of osteoarthritis. Paper presented at: 10th World Congress of the International Cartilage Repair Society; May 12-15, 2012; Montreal, Quebec, Canada.

21 Botter SM, van Osch GJVM, Clockaerts S, Waarsing JH, Weinans H, van Leeuwen JPTM. Osteoarthritis induction leads to early and temporal subchondral plate porosity in the tibial plateau of mice: an in vivo microfocal computed tomography study. *Arthritis Rheum*. 2011;63:2690-2699.

22 Weinans H, Siebelt M, Agricola R, Botter SM, Piscaer TM, Waarsing JH. Pathophysiology of peri-articular bone changes in osteoarthritis. *Bone*. 2012;51:190-196.

23 Kumarasinghe DD, Perilli E, Tsangari H, et al. Critical molecular regulators, histomorphometric indices and their correlations in the trabecular bone in primary hip osteoarthritis. *Osteoarthritis Cartilage*. 2010;18:1337-1344.

24 Sakao K, Takahashi KA, Arai Y, et al. Osteoblasts derived from osteophytes produce interleukin-6, interleukin-8, and matrix metalloproteinase-13 in osteoarthritis. *J Bone Miner Metab*. 2009;27:412-423.

25 Menkes C-J, Lane NE. Are osteophytes good or bad? *Osteoarthritis Cartilage*. 2004;12(suppl A):S53-S54.

26 Sellam J, Berenbaum F. The role of synovitis in pathophysiology and clinical symptoms of osteoarthritis. *Nat Rev Rheumatol*. 2010;6:625-635.

27 Scanzello CR, Goldring SR. The role of synovitis in osteoarthritis pathogenesis. *Bone*. 2012;51:249-257.

28 Hill CL, Seo GS, Gale D, Totterman S, Gale ME, Felson DT. Cruciate ligament integrity in osteoarthritis of the knee. *Arthritis Rheum*. 2005;52:794-799.

29 Hasegawa A, Otsuki S, Pauli C, et al. Anterior cruciate ligament changes in the human knee joint in aging and osteoarthritis. *Arthritis Rheum*. 2012;64:696-704.

30 Sharma L, Chmiel JS, Almagor O, et al. The role of varus and valgus alignment in the initial development of knee cartilage damage by MRI: the MOST Study. *Ann Rheum Dis*. 2012;epub ahead of print.

31 Arden N, Nevitt MC. Osteoarthritis: epidemiology. *Best Pract Res Clin Rheumatol*. 2006;20:3-25.

32 Conde J, Scotece M, Gómez R, Lopez V, Gómez-Reino JJ, Gualillo O. Adipokines and osteoarthritis: novel molecules involved in the pathogenesis and progression of disease. *Arthritis*. 2011; epub doi: 10.1155/2011/203901.

33 Anandacoomarasamy A, Leibman S, Smith G, et al. Weight loss in obese people has structure-modifying effects on medial but not on lateral knee articular cartilage. *Ann Rheum Dis*. 2012;71:26-32.

34 Leong DJ, Sun HB. Events in articular chondrocytes with aging. *Curr Osteoporos Rep*. 2011;9:196-201.

35 Shimada H, Sakakima H, Tsuchimochi K, et al. Senescence of chondrocytes in aging articular cartilage: GADD45β mediates p21 expression in association with C/EBPβ in senescence-accelerated mice. *Pathol Res Pract*. 2011;207:225-231.

36 Brandl A, Hartmann A, Bechmann V, Graf B, Nerlich M, Angele P. Oxidative stress induces senescence in chondrocytes. *J Orthop Res*. 2011;29:1114-1120.

37 Dai S-M, Shan Z-Z, Nakamura H, et al. Catabolic stress induces features of chondrocyte senescence through overexpression of caveolin 1: possible involvement of caveolin 1–induced down-regulation of articular chondrocytes in the pathogenesis of osteoarthritis. *Arthritis Rheum*. 2006;54:818-831.

38 Martin JA, Buckwalter JA. The role of chondrocyte senescence in the pathogenesis of osteoarthritis and in limiting cartilage repair. *J Bone Joint Surg Am*. 2003;85(suppl 2):106-110.

39 Nah S-S, Choi I-Y, Lee CK, et al. Effects of advanced glycation end products on the expression of COX-2, PGE_2 and NO in human osteoarthritic chondrocytes. *Rheumatology (Oxford)*. 2008;47:425-431.

40 Nah S-S, Choi I-Y, Yoo B, Kim YG, Moon H-B, Lee C-K. Advanced glycation end products increases matrix metalloproteinase-1, -3, and -13, and TNF-α in human osteoarthritic chondrocytes. *FEBS Lett.* 2007;581:1928-1932.

41 Huang C-Y, Lai K-Y, Hung L-F, Wu W-L, Liu F-C, Ho L-J. Advanced glycation end products cause collagen II reduction by activating Janus kinase/signal transducer and activator of transcription 3 pathway in porcine chondrocytes. *Rheumatology (Oxford).* 2011;50:1379-1389.

42 Hiran TS, Moulton PJ, Hancock JT. Detection of superoxide and NADPH oxidase in porcine articular chondrocytes. *Free Radic Biol Med.* 1997;23:736-743.

43 Tiku ML, Shah R, Allison GT. Evidence linking chondrocyte lipid peroxidation to cartilage matrix protein degradation. Possible role in cartilage aging and the pathogenesis of osteoarthritis. *J Biol Chem.* 2000;275:20069-20076.

44 Jallali N, Ridha H, Thrasivoulou C, Underwood C, Butler PEM, Cowen T. Vulnerability to ROS-induced cell death in ageing articular cartilage: the role of antioxidant enzyme activity. *Osteoarthritis Cartilage.* 2005;13:614-622.

45 Blanco F, Rego I, Ruiz-Romero C. The role of mitochondria in osteoarthritis. *Nat Rev Rheumatol.* 2011;7:161-169.

46 Loeser RF, Shanker G, Carlson CS, Gardin JF, Shelton BJ, Sonntag WE. Reduction in the chondrocyte response to insulin-like growth factor 1 in aging and osteoarthritis: studies in a non-human primate model of naturally occurring disease. *Arthritis Rheum.* 2000;43:2110-2120.

47 Martin JA, Ellerbroek SM, Buckwalter JA. Age-related decline in chondrocyte response to insulin-like growth factor-I: the role of growth factor binding proteins. *J Orthop Res.* 1997;15:491-498.

48 Chubinskaya S, Kumar B, Merrihew C, Heretis K, Rueger DC, Kuettner KE. Age-related changes in cartilage endogenous osteogenic protein-1 (OP-1). *Biochim Biophys Acta.* 2002;1588:126-134.

49 Blaney Davidson EN, Scharstuhl A, Vitters EL, van der Kraan PM, van den Berg WB. Reduced transforming growth factor-beta signaling in cartilage of old mice: role in impaired repair capacity. *Arthritis Res Ther.* 2005;7:R1338-R1347.

50 Scharstuhl A, van Beuningen HM, Vitters EL, van der Kraan PM, van den Berg WB. Loss of transforming growth factor counteraction on interleukin 1 mediated effects in cartilage of old mice. *Ann Rheum Dis.* 2002;61:1095-1098.

51 Loeser RF, Pacione CA, Chubinskaya S. The combination of insulin-like growth factor 1 and osteogenic protein 1 promotes increased survival of and matrix synthesis by normal and osteoarthritic human articular chondrocytes. *Arthritis Rheum.* 2003;48:2188-2196.

52 Lee SW, Song YS, Lee SY, et al. Downregulation of protein kinase CK2 activity facilitates tumor necrosis factor-α-mediated chondrocyte death through apoptosis and autophagy. *PLoS One.* 2011;6:e19163.

53 Taniguchi N, Caramés B, Ronfani L, et al. Aging-related loss of the chromatin protein HMGB2 in articular cartilage is linked to reduced cellularity and osteoarthritis. *Proc Natl Acad Sci USA.* 2009;106:1181-1186.

54 Scanzello CR, Plaas A, Crow MK. Innate immune system activation in osteoarthritis: is osteoarthritis a chronic wound? *Curr Opin Rheumatol.* 2008;20:565-572.

55 Goldring MB. Update on the biology of the chondrocyte and new approaches to treating cartilage diseases. *Best Pract Res Clin Rheumatol.* 2006;20:1003-1025.

56 Mobasheri A. Osteoarthritis 2012 year in review: biomarkers. *Osteoarthritis Cartilage.* 2012;20:1451-1464.

57 Henrotin Y, Gharbi M, Mazzucchelli G, Dubuc J-E, De Pauw E, Deberg M. Fibulin 3 peptides Fib3-1 and Fib3-2 are potential biomarkers of osteoarthritis. *Arthritis Rheum.* 2012;64:2260-2267.

58 Wang Y, Li D, Xu N, et al. Follistatin-like protein 1: a serum biochemical marker reflecting the severity of joint damage in patients with osteoarthritis. *Arthritis Res Ther.* 2011;13:R193.

59 Li D, Wang Y, Xu N, et al. Follistatin-like protein 1 is elevated in systemic autoimmune diseases and correlated with disease activity in patients with rheumatoid arthritis. *Arthritis Res Ther.* 2011;13:R17.

60 Lanyon P, O'Reilly S, Jones A, Doherty M. Radiographic assessment of symptomatic knee osteoarthritis in the community: definitions and normal joint space. *Ann Rheum Dis.* 1998;57:595-601.

61 Cicuttini FM, Baker J, Hart DJ, Spector TD. Association of pain with radiological changes in different compartments and views of the knee joint. *Osteoarthritis Cartilage.* 1996;4:143-147.

62 Felson DT, Chaisson CE, Hill CL, et al. The association of bone marrow lesions with pain in knee osteoarthritis. *Ann Intern Med.* 2001;134:541-549.

63 Xu L, Hayashi D, Roemer FW, Felson DT, Guermazi A. Magnetic resonance imaging of subchondral bone marrow lesions in association with osteoarthritis. *Semin Arthritis Rheum.* 2012;42:105-118.

Chapter 4
Clinical features and diagnosis of osteoarthritis

Francisco J. Blanco

Clinical criteria for osteoarthritis

Clinical criteria will continue to play an important role in the diagnosis of osteoarthritis until a diagnostic method that integrates clinical findings with aetiological, biochemical and histological abnormalities is developed [1]. One of the most enduring clinical criteria for osteoarthritis of the knee is the classification system developed for the American Rheumatism Association in 1986 [1]. The aim was to standardise and clarify the clinical definition of idiopathic osteoarthritis, using commonly available diagnostic techniques. This resulted in three sets of criteria, depending on whether the physician is able to draw on clinical examination and laboratory findings, clinical examination and radiographic results or clinical examination only (Table 4.1) [1].

Criteria for classification of idiopathic osteoarthritis of the knee

Clinical and laboratory	Clinical and radiographic	Clinical*
Knee pain + at least 5 of the following: • Age >50 years • Stiffness <30 minutes • Crepitus • Bony tenderness • Bony enlargement • No palpable warmth • ESR <40 mm/hour • RF <1:40 • SF OA	Knee pain + at least 1 of the following: • Age >50 years • Stiffness <30 minutes • Crepitus • Plus osteophytes	Knee pain + at least 3 of the following: • Age >50 years • Stiffness <30 minutes • Crepitus • Bony tenderness • Bony enlargement • No palpable warmth
92% sensitive, 75% specific	91% sensitive, 86% specific	95% sensitive, 69% specific

Table 4.1 Criteria for classification of idiopathic osteoarthritis of the knee. ESR, erythrocyte sedimentation rate (Westergren); RF, rheumatoid factor; SF OA, synovial fluid signs of osteoarthritis (clear, viscous or white blood cell count <2000/mm^3). *An alternative for the clinical category would be the presence of 4 of the 6 findings, which is 84% sensitive and 89% specific. Data from Altman et al [1]. Reproduced with permission from John Wiley and Sons.

A set of clinical definitions for knee osteoarthritis were also developed by Zhang et al for the European League Against Rheumatism (EULAR). The authors noted that, while radiography is often used as the 'gold standard' for diagnosis, it is not the only marker and the definition of knee osteoarthritis may change depending on the levels of care and clinical requirements [2]. They stated that a confident diagnosis can be made, without recourse to radiographic examination and even if radiographs appear normal, in adults aged >40 years with [2]:

- usage-related knee pain;
- only short-lived morning stiffness;
- functional limitation; and
- one or more typical examination findings (crepitus, restricted movement, bony enlargement).

The EULAR clinical criteria also emphasised that all patients with knee pain should be examined for possible osteoarthritis [2].

This publication has been made possible through an educational grant from SERVIER.

Symptoms of osteoarthritis

The onset of osteoarthritis symptoms is often insidious (Table 4.2) and there is often asymmetry of symptoms [3].

Symptoms and signs of osteoarthritis			
Symptoms		**Signs**	
Pain	Weakness	Joint (hard tissue) enlargement	Limitation of motion
Altered function	Deformity	Altered gait	Deformity
Stiffness	Grinding/clicking	Tenderness	Instability
Swelling	Instability/buckling	Crepitus	

Table 4.2 Symptoms and signs of osteoarthritis. The onset of symptoms of osteoarthritis is most often insidious, usually beginning in one or a few joints. Reproduced with permission from Altman [3].

Pain

Pain is the first and most predominant symptom of osteoarthritis [3–5] and is sometimes described as a deep ache [3]. The pain in weight-bearing joints is usually worsened by standing and walking is and relieved by rest. Although it is typically intermittent, pain can become constant [2,3]. The potential sites of origin for osteoarthritis pain are shown in Table 4.3 [3].

Pain in osteoarthritis: potential sites of origin	
Synovial inflammation	Outer one-third of menisci
Subchondral bone ischaemia ('bone angina')	Stress at ligamentous insertion
Distension of the joint capsule	Inflammation of bursae with/without calcification
Periarticular muscle spasm (eg, nocturnal myoclonus)	Osteophyte distension of periosteum or impingement of spinal canal/foramina

Table 4.3 Pain in osteoarthritis: potential sites of origin. The origin of pain in osteoarthritis is rarely clear, but sometimes can be attributed to anatomical changes in the joint. It is worth noting that there are no nerves in cartilage, the inner two-thirds of the menisci or synovial cavity. Hence, pain from these anatomic sites are induced indirectly through the above anatomical sites. Reproduced with permission from Altman [3]

In knee osteoarthritis, localised pain is often identified along the medial joint line or distal to the patellofemoral attachment. Medial pain is usually correlated with anatomic changes, as the medial compartment is involved in 70% of knee osteoarthritis cases [3]. In patients who have lateral compartment osteoarthritis, pain and grinding is localised to the lateral part of the knee and arthritic destruction is manifested as a valgus deformity [6].

Stiffness

Stiffness in osteoarthritis usually occurs in the morning, after periods of inactivity or especially in the evening [4]. The stiffness typically resolves within minutes and is relieved by motion of the joint [3], which distinguishes it from the prolonged stiffness (usually lasting over 30 minutes) experienced by rheumatoid arthritis sufferers [4].

Loss of movement or function

As osteoarthritis progresses, joint motion becomes restricted [3]. This results in loss of movement and function, which, alongside pain, is a major reason that patients visit their family doctor [4]. Loss of movement can lead to difficulties with certain daily activities, such as stair climbing, walking and doing household chores [4].

Other symptoms

Other signs and symptoms associated with osteoarthritis include joint enlargement due to joint effusion, bony swelling or both. Crepitus, defined as a sensation of crackling or crunching, is also commonly felt on passive or active movement of an affected joint [4].

Soft tissue contractures can result in varus (inward) or valgus (outward) knee deformity in osteoarthritis (Figure 4.1) and lead to joint instability [5,7,8]. Patients may also experience what is described as 'buckling', or spontaneous yielding of the quadriceps with knee flexion and giving way. This may be due to pain, fixed flexion contracture of the knee, quadriceps weakness and patellar problems such pain and dislocation [8].

Although not common in knee osteoarthritis, synovial effusions may be found along the medial joint margin and in the suprapatellar bursa. Distension due to synovial effusion can lead to knee flexion. Late signs include tenderness on palpation and pain on passive motion [3].

Valgus and varus knee deformities in osteoarthritis

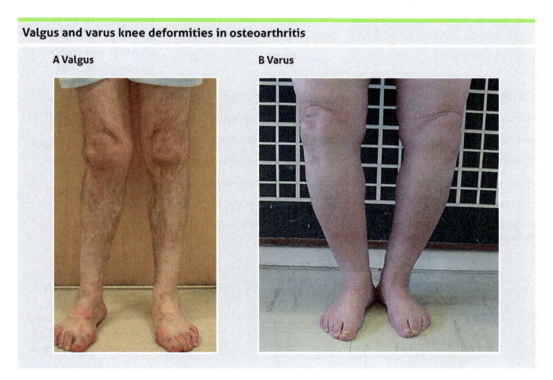

A Valgus   B Varus

Figure 4.1 Valgus and varus knee deformities in osteoarthritis.
A, This patient has a severe valgus deformity of the right knee and normal alignment of the left knee. Standing radiographs of his right knee showed changes indicative of osteoarthritis in the medial, lateral and patellofemoral compartments.
B, This patient has a severe varus deformity of both knees. Standing radiographs of her knees showed changes indicative of osteoarthritis in the medidal lateral and patellofemoral compartments. There is no cutaneous erythema to indicate the presence of acute inflammation in both knees, but the majority of specimens of synovial fluid aspirated from osteoarthritic knees contain crystals of either calcium pyrophosphate or apatite. Image courtesy of Dr FJ Blanco.

Effects on patient quality of life

Individuals with knee osteoarthritis have significantly poorer quality of life than healthy individuals, and pain affects all aspects of health-related quality of life (eg, sleep, mobility, energy) (Table 4.4) [9]. Furthermore, patients with proven osteoarthritis have lower function and pain scale scores than radiographically negative cases, indicating marked pain and worse functional status (Figure 4.2) [10].

Comparison of quality-of-life mean scores between patients with knee osteoarthritis and controls

	Knee osteoarthritis (mean ± SD) N=140	Control (mean ± SD) N=40	P value
Pain	74.66 ± 20.12	10.31 ± 10.16	<0.001
Energy level	51.38 ± 38.20	19.16 ± 22.50	<0.001
Emotional reaction	42.45 ± 31.31	9.68 ± 9.59	<0.001
Sleep	36.61 ± 26.72	15.50 ± 16.00	<0.001
Social isolation	19.14 ± 24.56	9.00 ± 10.07	<0.001
Physical mobility	42.72 ± 18.04	14.68 ± 8.43	<0.001

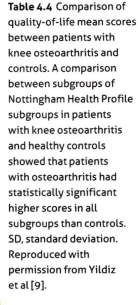

Table 4.4 Comparison of quality-of-life mean scores between patients with knee osteoarthritis and controls. A comparison between subgroups of Nottingham Health Profile subgroups in patients with knee osteoarthritis and healthy controls showed that patients with osteoarthritis had statistically significant higher scores in all subgroups than controls. SD, standard deviation. Reproduced with permission from Yildiz et al [9].

Studies have shown that patients with osteoarthritis also have a greater risk of mortality, particularly due to cardiovascular- and gastrointestinal-related causes. The decreased level of physical activity in those with walking disability probably contributes to the increased rate of cardiovascular death [11]. These findings were confirmed in a population-based cohort study of 1163 adults with osteoarthritis, which found higher rates of deaths in those studied than in the general population, especially for cardiovascular- and dementia-related mortality [12].

Scores and pain scales indicating marked pain and worse functional status

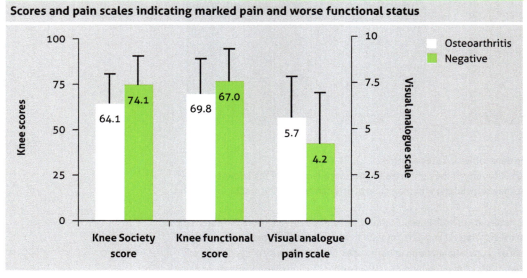

Figure 4.2 Scores and pain scales indicating marked pain and worse functional status. This figure shows Knee Society score, knee functional score and visual analogue pain scale in patients with proven osteoarthritis and radiographically negative cases. The patients with osteoarthritis had less favourable values than those who were radiographically negative. Reproduced with permission from Horváth et al [10].

Diagnosis of osteoarthritis

The primary goal of diagnostic evaluation is to either demonstrate the presence of osteoarthritis or to rule it out [13]. Osteoarthritis should always be suspected in patients who have joint-specific pain (typically usage-related) and loss of function [2,3], especially in the elderly [3].

Specific historical features of osteoarthritis

Pain	Pain at the beginning of movement	Permanent/nocturnal pain
	Pain during movement	Need for analgesics
Loss of function	Stiffness	Impairment in everyday activities
	Limitation of range of movement	Need for orthopaedic aids
Other symptoms	Crepitation	Stepwise progression
	Elevated sensitivity to cold and/or damp	

Table 4.5 Specific historical features of osteoarthritis. These historical criteria for osteoarthritis are those used at the Department of Orthopaedic and Trauma Surgery, University of Cologne. Reproduced with permission from Michael et al [13].

Risk factors, including age >50 years, female gender, high body mass index, previous knee injury or malalignment, joint laxity, occupational or recreational usage, family history and the presence of Heberden's nodes can help to identify patients in whom knee osteoarthritis is the most likely diagnosis [2].

Though not everyone with the signs and symptoms of osteoarthritis requires imaging studies, findings on plain radiograph can confirm the clinical findings. Nevertheless, only about 50% of patients with pathological or radiographic changes have symptoms [3].

While all patients with knee pain should be examined, the current 'gold standard' for morphological assessment of knee osteoarthritis is plain radiography [2]. The historical criteria for osteoarthritis that are relatively specific to the disorder are shown in Table 4.5, although they can be found in other joint diseases [13].

Differential diagnosis

While diagnosing osteoarthritis is easy, the primary difficulty is in knowing whether joint pain and disability are indeed due to the joint pathology that is characteristic of the disease [14]. Many patients with advanced pathology are asymptomatic and osteoarthritis pathology is extremely common in the elderly. Consequently, it cannot be assumed that symptomatic pain is due to osteoarthritis pathology in all individuals [14].

Pain may be referred, caused by periarticular problems (eg, bursitis due to ligamentous and meniscal lesions) or the result of pain sensitisation that leads to abnormal sensations with normal activities [2,14]. The involvement of other joints may suggest a range of alternative diagnoses, while severe local inflammation, erythema and progressive pain unrelated to usage may indicate crystals, sepsis or serious bone pathology [2]. Psychological factors such as depression and anxiety and social problems such as isolation can also play a role in pain development [14].

Physical examination

The physical findings of osteoarthritis are characteristic to each stage of the disorder [13]. Physical examinations should include all relevant tests, including inspection and palpation (Figure 4.3) [5], range of movement (Figure 4.4) [15] and special functional tests when required, such as meniscus tests, ligament stability and gait analysis [13]. Physical examination of the knee ligaments consists of [13]:

- testing of the lateral ligaments with varus or valgus stress; and
- testing of the anterior and posterior cruciate ligaments with the drawer test.

Knee examination and palpation

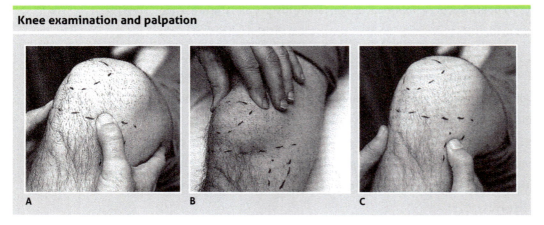

A   B   C

Figure 4.3 Knee examination and palpation.
A, Examination of the osteoarthritic knee should include palpation along and proximal to the joint line, indicated by the dashed line beneath the examiner's thumb. Crepitus can be elicited by passive flexion and extension of the joint. Palpation may reveal osteophytes that arise at the osteochondral margins or the joint or loose bodies. Tenderness in the gutters along the medial and lateral aspects of femoral condyles or in the suprapatellar bursa suggests underlying synovial inflammation. An estimate of the degree of medial-lateral laxity in the joint can be obtained by applying a valgus and then varus stress to the joint. **B**, Palpation of the margins of the patella, outlined here by the dashed circle below the examiner's fingers, may reveal osteophytes. The 'shrug sign', or knee pain produced by pressing above the patella (as illustrated), while the patient contracts the quadriceps muscle suggests that cartilage pathology is present in the patellofemoral portion of the knee.
C, Bursa palpation. The examiner's right thumb palpates the anserine bursa, which is below the knee and between the tibia and the pes anserine, a conjoint tendon of the sartorius and gracilis muscles that inserts on the proximal tibia. Pain that arises in the anserine bursa can mimic or exacerbate the pain of knee osteoarthritis and can be reproduced by deep palpation in this area. Local measures, such as hot packs or injection of the bursa with a mixture of bupivacaine and corticosteroids, usually are effective. Reproduced with permission from Myers [5].

The menisci should also be tested manually and the femoropatellar joint assessed for normal patellar mobility and indications of irritation [13].

Physical examination typically reveals evidence of mild-to-moderate tender swelling around the joint line, crepitus and restricted range of motion, with pain at the end of the range [14]. There may be tenderness over the joint line itself. Some patients can have evidence of mild inflammation, with warmth over the joint line and effusion. Joint deformities and instability may be seen in advanced cases [14].

Radiological methods in diagnosis

The most commonly used radiological method to confirm the clinical diagnosis of osteoarthritis is the plain radiograph [14], which can be used to establish the severity of joint damage and

Assessment for patellofemoral joint crepitation during active range of motion

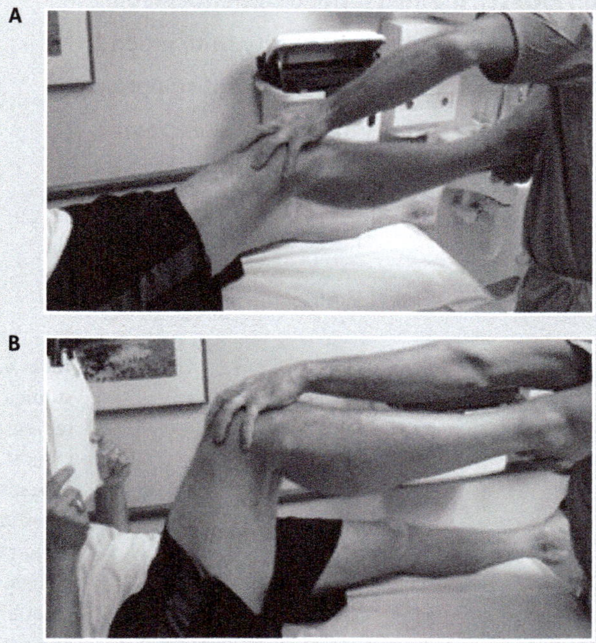

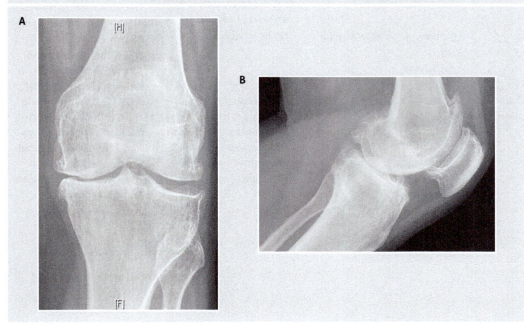

Figure 4.4 Assessment for patellofemoral joint crepitation during active range of motion. **A**, Extension. **B**, Flexion. Reproduced with permission from Griffith et al [15].

monitor disease progression [4,13]. Plain films should be obtained in a standardised manner in at least two planes: anteroposterior and lateral [13]. The main radiographic features associated with osteoarthritis are osteophytes, narrowing of the joint space due to articular cartilage loss and several changes in the subchondral bone, such as sclerosis, cysts, shape changes and loss of bone volume (Figure 4.5) [14].

Plain radiographs of a typical patient with severe osteoarthritis of the knee joint

Figure 4.5 Plain radiographs of a typical patient with severe osteoarthritis of the knee joint.
A, Note the loss of joint space, particularly marked in the medial compartment, caused by loss of articular cartilage, as well as the sclerosis of the underlying subchondral bone and osteophyte formation at the joint margin.
B, A lateral radiograph of the knee shows osteoarthritis in the patellofemoral compartment with large osteophytes. Image courtesy of Dr FJ Blanco.

There is a great deal of conflicting evidence about the relationship between radiographic findings and clinical symptoms (Table 4.6) [16–26]. However, the Kellgren and Lawrence grading system, which is based on radiographic findings, does reflect symptom severity, with grade 2 reflecting clinically important osteoarthritis [16]. One study noted a worsening of symptom severity between grades 1 and 2, with only a slight increase in severity between grades 0 and 1. It has been suggested that the worsening of symptoms between grades 2 and 3 is due to joint space narrowing, which is an important indicator of disease progression [16].

Summary of studies investigating radiographic findings and clinical symptoms in knee osteoarthritis

Study	N	Radiographs	Radiographic assessment	Clinical scales	Findings
Lanyon et al [21]	452	Standing AP, skyline	Osteophyte, JSN, subchondral sclerosis, cyst	Pain	Present correlation between osteophyte and knee pain, osteophyte as the best predictor for pain
Link et al [22]	50	AP, lateral, sunrise	KL grade	WOMAC	No correlation
McAlindon et al [23]	159	Standing AP, lateral	KL grade	Pain, disability (Stanford Health Assessment Questionnaire)	No correlation
Ozdemir et al [24]	84	Standing AP	Osteophyte, JSN	Range of motion	Correlation
Szebenyi et al [25]	167	Standing AP, lateral	KL grade	VAS pain score, WOMAC function	Structural changes in both compartments are correlated with pain and loss of function and subchondral sclerosis is associated with pain
Zhai et al [26]	500	Standing AP (semiflexed)	Osteophyte, JSN, subchondral sclerosis	WOMAC pain	No correlation
Cho et al [16]	600	Standing AP, 45° flexion PA, merchant	KL grade	WOMAC, SF-36	Correlation (+), women had more substantial symptomatic progression with increasing grades of knee osteoarthritis than men

Table 4.6 Summary of studies investigating radiographic findings and clinical symptoms in knee osteoarthritis. Although the relationship between radiographic findings and clinical symptoms in knee osteoarthritis has been examined, the worsening of symptoms by radiographic grade has not been well documented, especially in the general population. Many conflicting assertions have been made about the relationship between radiographic findings and clinical symptoms. AP, anteroposterior; JSN, joint space narrowing; KL, Kellgren and Lawrence; PA, posteroanterior; SF-36, short-form health survey (36 questions); VAS, visual analogue scale; WOMAC, Western Ontario and McMaster Universities Osteoarthritis Index. Data from [16–26]. Reproduced with permission from The Association of Bone and Joint Surgeons®.

Other imaging techniques are used to confirm an osteoarthritis diagnosis, such as computed tomography (CT), ultrasound and magnetic resonance imaging (MRI) (Table 4.7) [4]. While these modalities do not yield much additional diagnostic information, they can be used to assess the soft tissues and fluid-filled spaces (in the case of ultrasound) [10] or to exclude other diseases and conditions, including osteonecrosis (avascular necrosis), complex regional pain syndrome, Paget's disease, inflammatory arthropathies and stress fractures [4].

Imaging techniques for assessment of tissue-structure changes in osteoarthritis

Imaging technique	Primary use	Analyses	Advantages	Disadvantages
Plain radiograph*	Cartilage thickness	(Semi) quantitative	Low cost; easily applicable	Indirect, two-dimensional image of a three-dimensional problem
CT				
Standard*	Bone characteristics	Semiquantitative	3-dimensional	Radiation exposure, only bone
CECT	As standard plus cartilage volume	Semiquantitative	3-dimensional; information on cartilage	As standard plus contrast agent needed
MRI				
Standard SPGR*	Cartilage morphology	Quantitative	3-dimensional; quantitative	Time-consuming analyses
T2 MRI relaxation	Collagen distribution	Semiquantitative	Information on cartilage quality	Complex interpretation
T1ρ	Proteoglycan distribution	Semiquantitative	Information on cartilage quality	Complex interpretation
23Na MRI	FCD/ proteoglycan content	Semiquantitative	Information on cartilage quality	Field strength ≥3T
dGEMRIC	FCD/ proteoglycan content	Semiquantitative	Information on cartilage quality; early changes	Contrast agent needed
MRI whole-organ scoring				
KOSS	–	Semiquantitative	Whole-organ score	Time-consuming; observer variance
WORMS	–	Semiquantitative	Whole-organ score	Time-consuming; observer variance
BLOKS	–	Semiquantitative	Whole-organ score	Time-consuming; observer variance

Table 4.7 Imaging techniques for assessment of tissue-structure changes in osteoarthritis. *Techniques that have more common clinical and research applications for the assessment of cartilage (and bone), bone and synovial inflammation, as well as quantitative cartilage morphology (at present the most used magnetic resonance imaging [MRI] modality in clinical trials). BLOKS, Boston Leeds Osteoarthritis Knee score; CECT, contrast-enhanced computed tomography; CT, computed tomography; dGEMRIC, delayed gadolinium-enhanced MRI of cartilage; FCD, fixed charge density; KOSS, knee osteoarthritis scoring system; SPGR, spoiled gradient echo; WORMS, whole-organ MRI score. Reproduced with permission from Bijlsma et al [4].

Arthrocentesis

If palpable effusion is present, arthrocentesis, or the aspiration of synovial fluid, should be performed and the fluid analysed in order to rule out inflammatory disease and identify urate and calcium pyrophosphate crystals [2]. The fluid is typically viscous and translucent in comparison to aspirated fluid from a patient with rheumatoid arthritis, which is usually thinner and more opaque due to the greater number of inflammatory cells [14]. Osteoarthritis synovial fluid is usually non-inflammatory (<2000 leucocytes/mm³). Basic calcium phosphate crystals are also often present in synovial fluid [2].

Arthroscopy

Studies using arthroscopy, which is a minimally invasive technique [27], have found that approximately 50% of patients with osteoarthritis have localised proliferative changes and inflammatory changes of the synovium [28]. Moreover, macroscopic arthroscopy of the synovium appears to be more sensitive than weight-bearing radiographs in the detection of disease progression and may predict structural and clinical changes more accurately [28,29]. Arthroscopy can also be used to differentiate normal from reactive and inflammatory synovia in osteoarthritis (Table 4.8) [28,30,31], which may be an important distinction as synovial inflammation appears to have a direct effect on adjacent cartilage [31].

Arthroscopic features of synovial tissue

Synovial stage	Arthroscopic features
Normal synovium	Few translucent, slender villi with a fine vascular network can be clearly seen
	Proliferation of opaque villi
Reactive synovium	Villi have normal morphology or somewhat thicker and squat ('cut grass') appearance
	Vascular network not seen due to loss of translucence
Inflammatory synovium	Hypervascularisation of synovial membrane and/or proliferation of hypertrophic and hyperaemic villi are apparent

Table 4.8 Arthroscopic features of synovial tissue. Standardised macroscopic description established by Ayral et al [28,30] for the arthroscopic evaluation of the medial perimeniscal synovium. Data from Sellam & Berenbaum [31]. Reproduced with permission from Nature Publishing Group.

Staging of osteoarthritis

As osteoarthritis progresses, the clinical symptoms and signs and their radiological correlates follow a typical course, which can be incorporated into a clinically useful staging system. Several staging systems have been developed that vary in their weighting of subjective and objective criteria [13]. The Kellgren and Lawrence system, which has become the de facto standard for assessing osteoarthritis, is based on the typical signs of knee osteoarthritis seen on plain radiological films (Table 4.9) [32]. However, the Western Ontario and McMaster Universities Osteoarthritis Index (WOMAC) reflects the severity of the disease and allows a valid, reproducible assessment of the impairment caused by pain and loss of function [13,33,34]. While WOMAC is not commonly used in clinical practice [13], it is extensively used in clinical trials [35].

Kellgren and Lawrence staging system of knee osteoarthritis

Stage	Description
0	No abnormality
1	Incipient osteoarthritis, beginning of osteophyte formation on eminences
2	Moderate joint space narrowing, moderate subchondral sclerosis
3	>50% joint space narrowing, rounded femoral condyle, extensive subchondral sclerosis, extensive osteophyte formation
4	Joint destruction, obliterated joint space, subchondral cysts in the tibial head and femoral condyle, subluxed position

Table 4.9 Kellgren and Lawrence staging system of knee osteoarthritis. The typical radiological signs of knee osteoarthritis that can be seen on plain films are incorporated into the Kellgren and Lawrence staging system. Adapted from Kellgren & Lawrence [32]. Reproduced with permission from BMJ Publishing Group Ltd and the European League Against Rheumatism.

Osteoarthritis in other joints

While osteoarthritis is commonly manifested in the knee, it is also often seen in other joints, primarily in the hip and hand.

Hip osteoarthritis

Mechanical stresses to the hip over time, combined with biochemical alterations of cartilage can result in cartilage disruption. Eventually, this can lead to associated changes in subchondral bone, synovium, joint margins and para-articular structures that are the manifestations of hip osteoarthritis [36]. Figure 4.6 shows some of the joint changes seen with hip osteoarthritis. The superior pole is the most common area affected by hip osteoarthritis [14]. Pain may also be felt in the inguinal area, trochanter or along the tensor fascia lata [3]. Hip osteoarthritis is often closely linked with knee osteoarthritis [10].

Plain radiograph of osteoarthritic hip joints

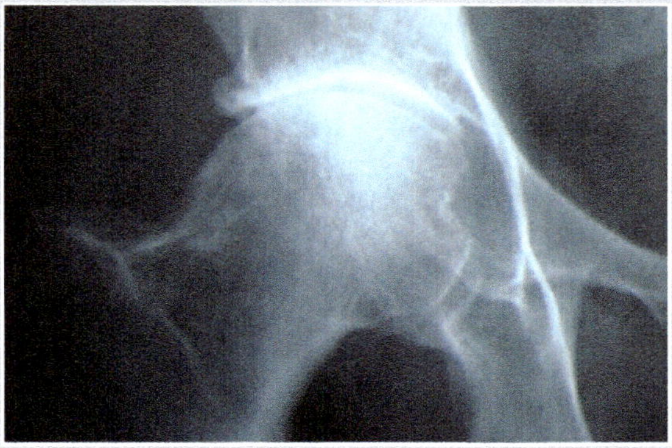

Figure 4.6 Plain radiograph of an osteoarthritic hip joint. Narrowing of the joint space, subchondral sclerosis and visible osteophythes can be seen in right hip. Image courtesy of Dr FJ Blanco.

Patients with hip osteoarthritis experience a gradual loss of range of motion, particularly internal and extension rotation [3]. This leads to a change in gait, which in the elderly contributes to an increase in falls. One study found that 45% of people aged ≥65 years with hip osteoarthritis had fallen at least once during a 12-month period, compared with the estimated general prevalence rate of 30% [37].

Classification criteria for hip osteoarthritis are given in Table 4.10 and can be used to rule out other causes of hip pain, such as spondyloarthropathy or rheumatoid arthritis [36].

Combined clinical and radiographical classification for osteoarthritis of the hip

Hip pain + at least 2 of the following:
Erythrocyte sedimentation rate <20 mm/hour
Radiographic femoral or acetabular osteophytes
Radiographic joint space narrowing (superior, axial and/or medial)

Table 4.10 Combined clinical and radiographical classification for osteoarthritis of the hip. This classification method yields a sensitivity of 89% and a specificity of 91%. Data from Altman et al [36]. Reproduced with permission from John Wiley and Sons.

Hand osteoarthritis

Hand osteoarthritis is primarily manifested as pain and swelling in the distal interphalangeal joints (Heberden's nodes), proximal interphalangeal joints (Bouchard's nodes) and thumb base joints [14,38]. There is often bony enlargement with or without deformity. Patients with polyarticular hand osteoarthritis are at greater risk of developing osteoarthritis in other sites [38].

Table 4.11 lists classification criteria for hand osteoarthritis [39]. Zhang et al have also developed clinical definitions for hand osteoarthritis for EULAR, as they felt that it merited its own recommendations. Similar to their recommendations for knee osteoarthritis diagnosis, they stated that a confident clinical diagnosis can be made in adults aged >40 years with [38]:

- pain on usage;
- intermittent symptoms; and
- only mild morning or inactivity stiffness affecting one or a few joints at any given time.

Combined clinical and radiographical classification for osteoarthritis of the hand
Hand pain, aching or stiffness + 3 or 4 of the following:
Hard tissue enlargement of 2 or more of 10 selected joints
Hard tissue enlargement of 2 or more DIP joints
Fewer than 3 swollen MCP joints
Deformity of at least 1 of 10 selected joints

Table 4.11 Combined clinical and radiographical classification for osteoarthritis of the hand. The 10 selected joints are the second and third distal interphalangeal (DIP), the second and third proximal interphalangeal and the first carpometacarpal joints of both hands. This classification method yields a sensitivity of 94% and a specificity of 87%. MCP, metacarpophalangeal. Data from Altman et al [39]. Reproduced with permission from John Wiley and Sons.

All of these criteria can be used to distinguish hand osteoarthritis from similar conditions such as rheumatoid arthritis, psoriatic arthritis or gout [38].

As with knee osteoarthritis, plain radiographs are the main method for conducting radiological assessments of hand osteoarthritis. Usually, posteroanterior radiographs of both hands are sufficient to make a diagnosis; features seen include joint space narrowing, subchondral bone sclerosis and subchondral cysts [38].

References

1   Altman R, Asch E, Bloch D, et al. Development of criteria for the classification and reporting of osteoarthritis. Classification of osteoarthritis of the knee. Diagnostic and Therapeutic Criteria Committee of the American Rheumatism Association. *Arthritis Rheum.* 1986;29:1039-1049.

2   Zhang W, Doherty M, Peat G, et al. EULAR evidence-based recommendations for the diagnosis of knee osteoarthritis. *Ann Rheum Dis.* 2010;69:483-489.

3   Altman RD. Osteoarthritis in the elderly population. In: Nakasato Y, Yung RL, eds. *Geriatric Rheumatology: A Comprehensive Approach.* New York, NY: Springer Science+Business Media, LLC; 2011:187-196.

4   Bijlsma JWJ, Berenbaum F, Lafeber FPJG. Osteoarthritis: an update with relevance for clinical practice. *Lancet.* 2011;377:2115-2126.

5   Myers SL. Osteoarthritis and crystal-associated synovitis. In: Hunder GG, ed. *Atlas of Rheumatology.* 4th ed. Philadelphia, PA: Current Medicine LLC; 2005:54-81.

6   Bal BS, Lavernia CJ. Surgical treatment of lateral compartment arthritis. Available at: emedicine. medscape.com/article/1251688-overview. Accessed December 5, 2012.

7   Engh GA. The difficult knee: severe varus and valgus. *Clin Orthop Relat Res.* 2003;416:58-63.

8   Vince KG, Abdeen A, Sugimori T. The unstable total knee arthroplasty: causes and cures. *J Arthroplasty*. 2006;21(4 suppl 1):44-49.

9   Yildiz N, Topuz O, Gungen GO, Deniz S, Alkan H, Ardic F. Health-related quality of life (Nottingham Health Profile) in knee osteoarthritis: correlation with clinical variables and self-reported disability. *Rheumatol Int*. 2010;30:1595-1600.

10   Horváth G, Koroknai G, Ács B, Than P, Bellyei Á, Illés T. Prevalence of radiographic primary hip and knee osteoarthritis in a representative central European population. *Int Orthop*. 2011;35:971-975.

11   Hochberg MC. Mortality in osteoarthritis. *Clin Exp Rheumatol*. 2008;26(suppl 51):S120-S124.

12   Nüesch E, Dieppe P, Reichenbach S, Williams S, Iff S, Jüni P. All cause and disease specific mortality in patients with knee or hip osteoarthritis: population based cohort study. *BMJ*. 2011;342:d1165.

13   Michael JW-P, Schlüter-Brust KU, Eysel P. The epidemiology, etiology, diagnosis, and treatment of osteoarthritis of the knee. *Dtsch Arztebl Int*. 2010;107:152-162.

14   Dieppe P. Osteoarthritis. A. Clinical features In: Klippel JH, Stone JH, Crofford LJ, White PH, eds. *Primer on the Rheumatic Diseases*. 13th ed. New York, NY: Springer Science+Business Media, LLC; 2008:224-228.

15   Griffith CJ, LaPrade RF. Medial plica irritation: diagnosis and treatment. *Curr Rev Musculoskelet Med*. 2008;1:53-60.

16   Cho HJ, Chang CB, Yoo JH, Kim SJ, Kim TK. Gender differences in the correlation between symptom and radiographic severity in patients with knee osteoarthritis. *Clin Orthop Relat Res*. 2010;468:1749-1758.

17   Barker K, Lamb SE, Toye F, Jackson S, Barrington S. Association between radiographic joint space narrowing, function, pain and muscle power in severe osteoarthritis of the knee. *Clin Rehabil*. 2004;18:793-800.

18   Bruyere O, Honore A, Rovati LC, et al. Radiologic features poorly predict clinical outcomes in knee osteoarthritis. *Scand J Rheumatol*. 2002;31:13-16.

19   Cicuttini FM, Baker J, Hart DJ, Spector TD. Association of pain with radiological changes in different compartments and views of the knee joint. *Osteoarthritis Cartilage*. 1996;4:143-147.

20   Dieppe PA, Cushnaghan J, Shepstone L. The Bristol 'OA500' study: progression of osteoarthritis (OA) over 3 years and the relationship between clinical and radiographic changes at the knee joint. *Osteoarthritis Cartilage*. 1997;5:87-97.

21   Lanyon P, O'Reilly S, Jones A, Doherty M. Radiographic assessment of symptomatic knee osteoarthritis in the community: definitions and normal joint space. *Ann Rheum Dis*. 1998;57:595-601.

22   Link TM, Steinbach LS, Ghosh S, et al. Osteoarthritis: MR imaging findings in different stages of disease and correlation with clinical findings. *Radiology*. 2003;226:373-381.

23   McAlindon TE, Cooper C, Kirwan JR, Dieppe PA. Determinants of disability in osteoarthritis of the knee. *Ann Rheum Dis*. 1993;52:258-262.

24   Ozdemir F, Tukenmez O, Kokino S, Turan FN. How do marginal osteophytes, joint space narrowing and range of motion affect each other in patients with knee osteoarthritis. *Rheumatol Int*. 2006;26:516-522.

25   Szebenyi B, Hollander AP, Dieppe P, et al. Associations between pain, function, and radiographic features in osteoarthritis of the knee. *Arthritis Rheum*. 2006;54:230-235.

26   Zhai G, Blizzard L, Srikanth V, et al. Correlates of knee pain in older adults: Tasmanian Older Adult Cohort Study. *Arthritis Rheum*. 2006;55:264-271.

27   af Klint E, Catrina AI, Matt P, et al. Evaluation of arthroscopy and macroscopic scoring. *Arthritis Res Ther*. 2009;11:R81.

28   Ayral X, Pickering EH, Woodworth TG, Mackillop N, Dougados M. Synovitis: a potential predictive factor of structural progression of medial tibiofemoral knee osteoarthritis – results of a 1 year longitudinal arthroscopic study in 422 patients. *Osteoarthritis Cartilage*. 2005;13:361-367.

29   Ayral X. Efficacy and role of topical treatment of gonarthrosis. *Presse Med*. 1999;28:1195-1200.

30   Ayral X, Mayoux-Benhamou A, Dougados M. Proposed scoring system for assessing synovial membrane abnormalities at arthroscopy in knee osteoarthritis. *Br J Rheumatol*. 1996;35 (suppl 3):14-17.

31   Sellam J, Berenbaum F. The role of synovitis in pathophysiology and clinical symptoms of osteoarthritis. *Nat Rev Rheumatol*. 2010;6:625-635.

32   Kellgren JH, Lawrence JS. Radiological assessment of osteo-arthrosis. *Ann Rheum Dis*. 1957;16:494-502.

33   Bellamy N, Buchanan WW, Goldsmith CH, Campbell J, Stitt LW. Validation study of WOMAC: a health status instrument for measuring clinically important patient relevant outcomes to antirheumatic drug therapy in patients with osteoarthritis of the hip or knee. *J Rheumatol*. 1988;15:1833-1840.

34 Bellamy N. WOMAC Osteoarthritis Index. WOMAC® 3.1 Index. Available at: www.womac.com. Accessed March 5, 2013.

35 American College of Rheumatology. Western Ontario and McMaster Universities Osteoarthritis Index (WOMAC). Available at: www.rheumatology.org/practice/clinical/clinicianresearchers/outcomes-instrumentation/WOMAC.asp. Accessed December 4, 2012.

36 Altman R, Alarcón G, Appelrouth D, et al. The American College of Rheumatology criteria for the classification and reporting of osteoarthritis of the hip. *Arthritis Rheum.* 1991;34:505-514.

37 Arnold CM, Faulkner RA. The history of falls and the association of the timed up and go test to falls and near-falls in older adults with hip osteoarthritis. *BMC Geriatr.* 2007;7:17.

38 Zhang W, Doherty M, Leeb BF, et al. EULAR evidence-based recommendations for the diagnosis of hand osteoarthritis: report of a task force of ESCISIT. *Ann Rheum Dis.* 2009;68:8-17.

39 Altman R, Alarcón G, Appelrouth D, et al. The American College of Rheumatology criteria for the classification and reporting of osteoarthritis of the hand. *Arthritis Rheum.* 1990;33:1601-1610.

Chapter 5
Assessing joint damage in osteoarthritis

Daichi Hayashi, Frank W. Roemer and Ali Guermazi

Introduction

Osteoarthritis is a highly prevalent joint disease that primarily affects the elderly (see Figures 2.4 and 2.5). The increasing importance of imaging in osteoarthritis for diagnosis, prognostication and follow-up is well recognised by clinicians and osteoarthritis researchers. While conventional radiography is the gold standard imaging technique for the evaluation of known or suspected osteoarthritis in clinical practice and research, it has limitations that have become apparent in the course of recent magnetic resonance imaging (MRI)-based knee osteoarthritis studies [1]. Of the common imaging techniques, only MRI can assess all of the structures of the joint (ie, cartilage, meniscus, subarticular bone marrow and synovium) (Table 5.1), and thus can show the knee as a whole organ three-dimensionally and directly help in the assessment of cartilage morphology and composition. This imaging modality, therefore, plays a crucial role in increasing our understanding of the natural history of osteoarthritis and in the development of new therapies. The uses and the limitations of conventional radiography, MRI and other techniques such as ultrasound, nuclear medicine, computed tomography (CT) and CT arthrography in the imaging of osteoarthritis in both clinical practice and research are described in this chapter.

Pathological features that can be visualised by radiography and magnetic resonance imaging in osteoarthritis-affected joints

Radiography	MRI
Osteophytes	Osteophytes
Subchondral cysts	Subchondral, intraarticular and periarticular cysts
Sclerosis	Cartilage loss
Joint space narrowing/loss	Bone marrow oedema pattern (bone marrow lesion)
Malalignment of the joint	Attrition
	Effusion
	Synovitis (with contrast-enhanced magnetic resonance imaging)
	Ligamentous lesions
	Meniscal damage/extrusion (knee)
	Labral lesions (shoulder and hip)
	Intervertebral disc pathology (spine)

Table 5.1 Pathological features that can be visualised by radiography and magnetic resonance imaging in osteoarthritis-affected joints.

This publication has been made possible through an educational grant from SERVIER.

N. Arden et al., *Atlas of Osteoarthritis*, DOI 10.1007/978-1-910315-16-3_5,
© Springer Healthcare 2014

Conventional radiography

It is common to acquire knee radiographs in the posteroanterior fixed-flexion view using the SynaFlexer™ (Synarc Inc., Boston, MA, USA) positioning frame. This method permits highly fairly precise and reproducible measurements of joint space width. Radiographically, osteoarthritis is defined as the presence of definite osteophytes [2]. An increase in joint space narrowing (JSN) is the most commonly used criterion for assessing the progression of osteoarthritis, and the complete loss of joint space width characterised by bone-on-bone contact is an indicator for joint replacement. Currently, radiographically detected JSN is the only US Food and Drug Administrator- and European Medicines Agency-recommended imaging-based end point for phase III osteoarthritis clinical trials. The low cost and wide availability makes radiography the first choice of imaging for routine clinical management of osteoarthritis patients.

Radiography enables the detection of bony features associated with osteoarthritis, including marginal osteophytes, subchondral sclerosis, attrition and subchondral cysts (Figure 5.1). The presence of these features can be observed in any joint affected by osteoarthritis. Loss of joint space is an indirect marker of articular cartilage loss because it is not possible to directly

---

Radiographic manifestations of osteoarthritis

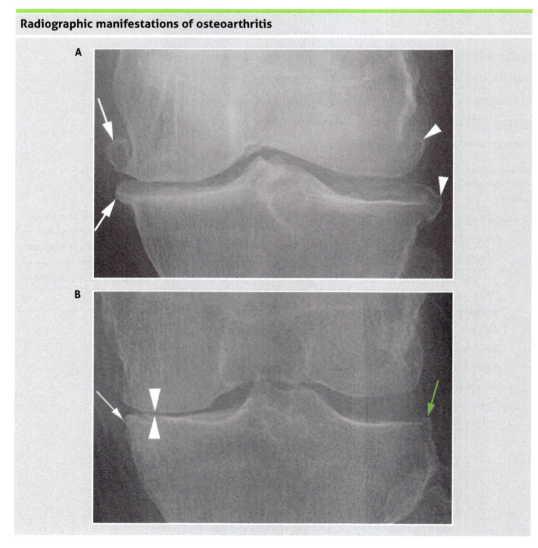

Figure 5.1 Radiographic manifestations of osteoarthritis. **A**, Anteroposterior (AP) radiograph of the knee shows large marginal osteophytes of the medial (arrows) and lateral (arrowheads) tibiofemoral compartments. Note additional joint space narrowing (JSN) of the medial compartment. Image represents the hypertrophic phenotype of tibiofemoral osteoarthritis with severe osteophyte formation and comparatively discrete JSN. **B**, Atrophic phenotype of osteoarthritis. AP radiograph of the knee shows severe JSN of the medial compartment (arrowheads). Only tiny osteophytes are seen at the medial (white arrow) and lateral (green arrow) joint margins. Figure courtesy of Drs D Hayashi, FW Roemer and A Guermazi.

visualise cartilage on radiographs. In the knee joint, radiographic joint space width reflects both cartilage thickness and meniscal integrity, but precise measurement of these articular structures is impossible with radiography.

The severity of osteoarthritis can be semiquantitatively assessed using published scoring systems. In the most widely utilised system, the Kellgren and Lawrence (KL) grade, the presence of radiographic osteoarthritis is defined as KL grade 2 or above [3]. However, KL grading has limitations; for example, KL grade 3 includes all degrees of JSN, regardless of actual extent (Figure 5.2). By contrast, the Osteoarthritis Research Society International classification grades tibiofemoral joint space width and osteophytes separately for each compartment of the knee [4]. Compartmental scoring appears to be more sensitive to longitudinal radiographic changes than KL grading [1]. Joint space width can also be assessed quantitatively using a ruler, either a physical device or a software application, to measure the joint space width as the distance between the projected femoral and tibial margins on the image. Joint space width is highly dependent on the angulation and positioning of the knee joint at the time of radiographic acquisition, and thus the use of a positioning frame (such as the SynaFlexer™) is important in regard to the reproducibility of measurements. Progression of JSN is a known predictor of knee replacement surgery at a later stage of life.

Insensitivity of semiquantitative assessment of radiographic joint space narrowing

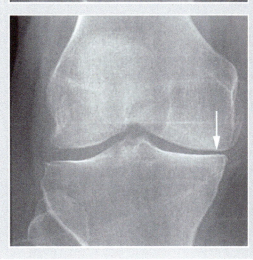

Figure 5.2 Insensitivity of semiquantitative assessment of radiographic joint space narrowing. **A**, Anteroposterior radiograph of the knee shows definite joint space narrowing (JSN) of the medial tibiofemoral compartment (arrowhead). This represents grade 3 tibiofemoral osteoarthritis according to the Kellgren and Lawrence (KL) grading scheme. **B**, Two years later, there is definite worsening of JSN, but still no bone-to-bone contact. This will still be scored as grade 3 according to KL scheme. Semiquantitative scoring has only a limited capacity for assessing progression in KL grade 3 osteoarthritis. Figure courtesy of Drs D Hayashi, FW Roemer and A Guermazi.

Magnetic resonance imaging

Magnetic resonance imaging can depict all components of the joint (Table 5.1, Figures 5.3 and 5.4), allowing for the joint to be evaluated as a whole organ. In general, fluid-sensitive fat-suppressed sequences (eg, T2-weighted, proton density-weighted or intermediate-weighted fast spin echo sequences) are useful for evaluating cartilage, bone marrow, ligaments, menisci and tendons [5]. These sequences are essential to assess focal cartilage defects and bone marrow

Superiority of magnetic resonance imaging for depicting osteoarthritis as a whole-joint disease

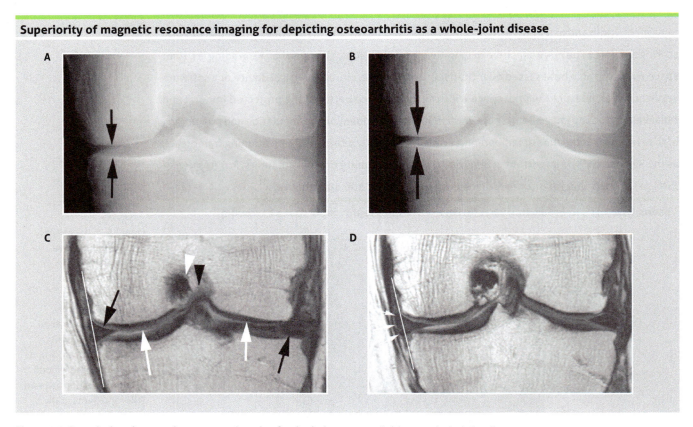

Figure 5.3 Superiority of magnetic resonance imaging for depicting osteoarthritis as a whole-joint disease.
A, Baseline anteroposterior radiograph shows normal medial tibiofemoral joint space width (arrows).
B, At the 3-year follow-up, definite joint space narrowing (JSN) is detected. Soft tissues are not visible on the radiograph.
C, Baseline magnetic resonance image (MRI) of the same knee shows multiple tissues relevant to osteoarthritis that are not depicted by the radiograph. Cartilage is visualised indirectly as a structure of intermediate signal intensity in this proton density-weighted coronal MRI (white arrows). The anterior (white arrowhead) and posterior (black arrowhead) cruciate ligaments are clearly depicted as hypointense structures. In addition, the menisci are visualised as hypointense triangular structures in the medial and lateral joint space (black arrows). Note that the medial meniscus is aligned with the medial joint margin (white line).
D, At the 3-year follow-up, the MRI shows incident meniscal extrusion of the medial meniscal body, which is responsible for the radiographic JSN (arrowheads and white line). No cartilage loss is observed during the follow-up interval. Figure courtesy of Drs D Hayashi, FW Roemer and A Guermazi.

Spine osteoarthritis

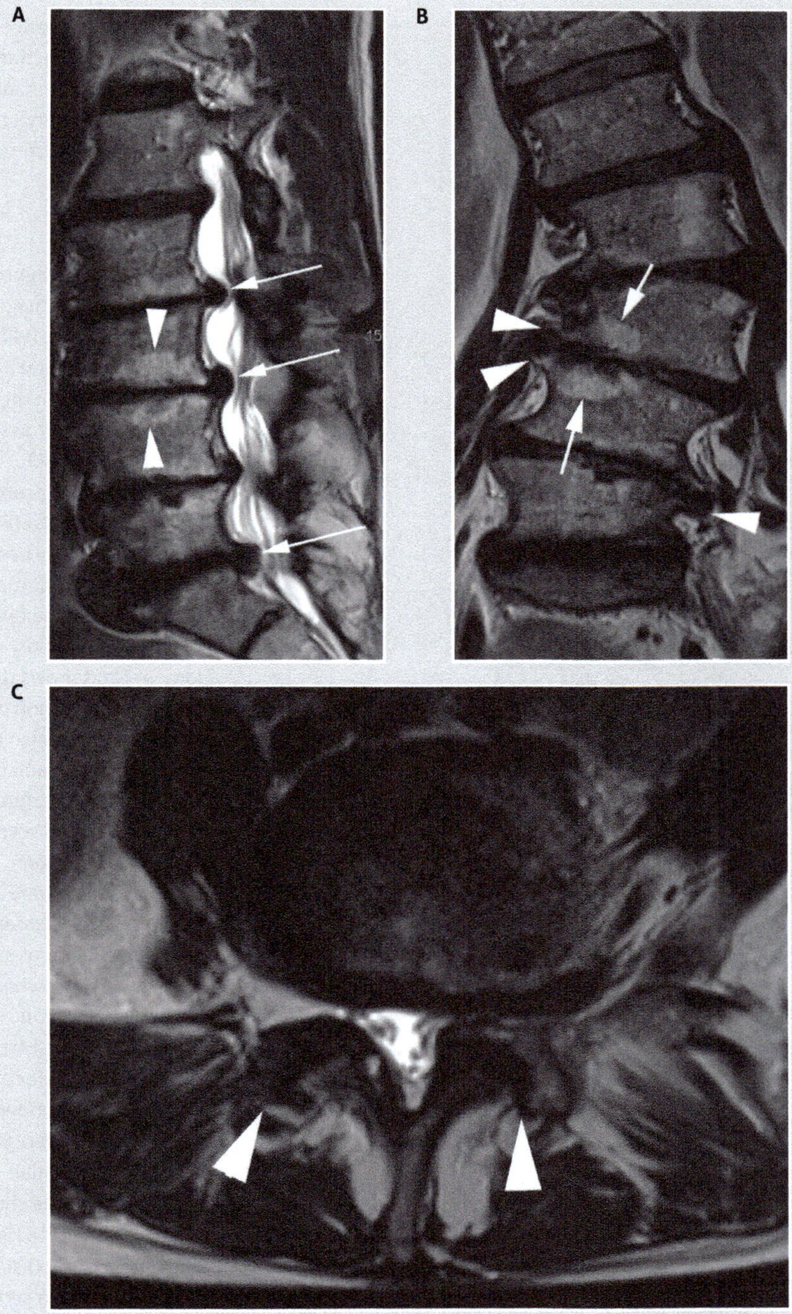

Figure 5.4 Spine osteoarthritis. **A**, Sagittal T2-weighted magnetic resonance image shows severe degenerative changes of the lumbar spine. There is marked narrowing of the intervertebral spaces L2–S1 with adjacent bone marrow alterations reflecting lipomatous endplate conversion (arrowheads). In addition, severe disc bulging is observed, leading to spinal canal stenosis (arrows). **B**, Corresponding coronal T2-weighted image shows severe left-convex scoliosis and marginal osteophyte formation (arrowheads). Circumscribed fatty peridiscal endplate changes in the L3/4 segment are seen (arrows). **C**, Corresponding T2-weighted axial image shows severe hypertrophic facet joint osteoarthritis (arrowheads), causing spinal canal stenosis in conjunction with ligamentum flavum hypertrophy and disc bulging. Figure courtesy of Drs D Hayashi, FW Roemer and A Guermazi.

lesions. Gradient recalled echo-type sequences (eg, 3-dimensional spoiled gradient echo at steady state and double echo steady state) are not suitable for assessing marrow or focal defects as they are prone to susceptibility artefacts, which hinder accurate interpretation (Figures 5.5 and 5.6; see pages 72 and 73) [6]. However, these sequences provide high spatial resolution and excellent contrast of cartilage to subchondral bone and are well suited for quantitative measurement of volume and thickness based on segmentation [7]. For the assessment of synovitis, only contrast-enhanced MRI can depict the true extent of synovial thickening and thus is preferable to noncontrast-enhanced MRI [8].

Relevance of sequence selection for magnetic resonance imaging assessment of different osteoarthritis features

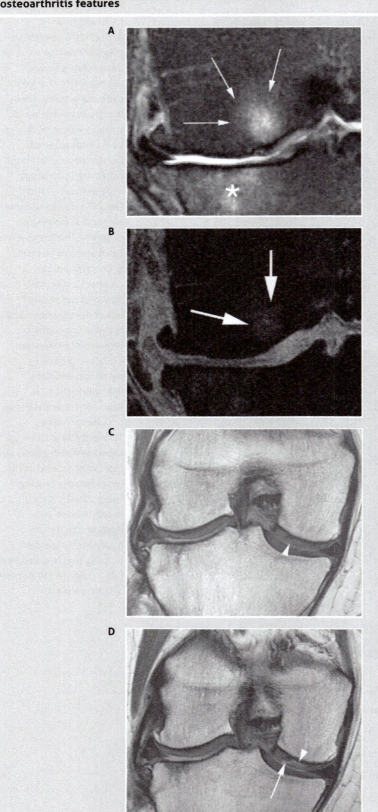

Figure 5.5 Relevance of sequence selection for magnetic resonance imaging assessment of different osteoarthritis features. **A**, This coronal fat-suppressed, intermediate-weighted, turbo-spin echo magnetic resonance image (MRI) shows subchondral bone marrow lesions in the medial femur (arrows) and tibia (asterisk). **B**, Corresponding coronal fast low angle shot (FLASH) image, commonly used for cartilage segmentation, barely depicts the femoral bone marrow lesion (arrows) and shows tibial bone marrow lesion only minimally. Note also the marked femoral and tibial cartilage loss, marginal osteophytes and severe meniscal extrusion. **C**, At baseline, a very discrete surface indentation of the cartilaginous surface is observed (arrowhead). **D**, At the 2-year follow-up, a definite fissure-like, full-thickness defect has developed that undermines the chondral coverage representing partial delamination. The chondral fragment is at high risk of detaching. **C** and **D** show development of a small focal cartilage defect over 2 years as visualised by intermediate-weighted MRI, which is ideally suited to depicting these early focal cartilage surface changes. Figure courtesy of Drs D Hayashi, FW Roemer and A Guermazi.

Artefacts on magnetic resonance imaging

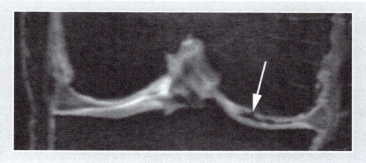

Figure 5.6 Artefacts on magnetic resonance imaging. Coronal dual-echo steady-state image shows a hypointense linear finding in the medial tibiofemoral joint space. The so-called vacuum phenomenon is responsible for this artefact, which can easily be mistaken for a solid structure. Assessment of the articular surface is impaired and signal loss within the cartilaginous contour must not be mistaken for a surface lesion (arrow). Figure courtesy of Drs D Hayashi, FW Roemer and A Guermazi.

Ultrasound

Ultrasound enables multiplanar and real-time imaging, but it has limitations. Ultrasound imaging is a manual process, not a semi-automated process like other imaging modalities and is operator-dependent; ie, the quality of image acquired can vary depending on who is performing the scanning. An experienced and skilled radiologist/sonographer can produce much better quality images than someone who is less skilled. Also, the planes obtained may vary from one operator to another independent of their experience, rendering comparison of multiple examinations very difficult. Another limitation of ultrasound is that it cannot assess deep intraarticular structures or subchondral bone.

The major advantage of ultrasound over radiography is its ability to detect synovial pathology (Figure 5.7). Ultrasound is also more sensitive than clinical examination in detecting synovial hypertrophy and joint effusion [9]. Additionally, colour-coded Doppler signal has been validated as an indirect measure of histological synovial vascularity in large joint osteoarthritis [10]. Articular cartilage and the meniscus can be imaged with ultrasound [11,12], and in hand osteoarthritis, ultrasound can be used to monitor the efficacy of corticosteroid injection therapy for synovitis [13].

Ultrasound image of the medial tibiofemoral joint space in advanced osteoarthritis

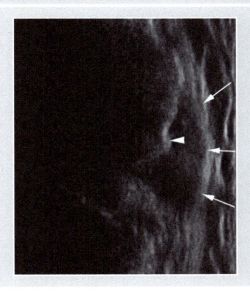

Figure 5.7 Ultrasound image of the medial tibiofemoral joint space in advanced osteoarthritis. Image shows marked extrusion of the body of the medial meniscus (arrows). In addition, a small femoral osteophyte is depicted (arrowhead). Note the sound extinction toward the more central parts of the joint (left in the image), which makes assessment of the cartilage surface and the ligaments in these areas of the joint impossible. Figure courtesy of Drs D Hayashi, FW Roemer and A Guermazi.

Computed tomography and computed tomography arthrography

Computed tomography is a valuable tool when imaging of osseous changes or detailed pre-surgical planning is required. It depicts cortical bone and soft tissue calcifications better than MRI (Figure 5.8) and has an established clinical role in assessing facet-joint osteoarthritis of the spine [14]. CT arthrography is an alternative method for indirect visualisation of cartilage and other intrinsic joint structures, especially in the knee and shoulder joints, and it enables imaging of focal cartilage defects (Figure 5.9) [15]. Penetration of contrast medium within deeper layers of the cartilage surface indicates an articular-sided defect of the chondral surface.

Use of computed tomography for evaluation of osteoarthritis

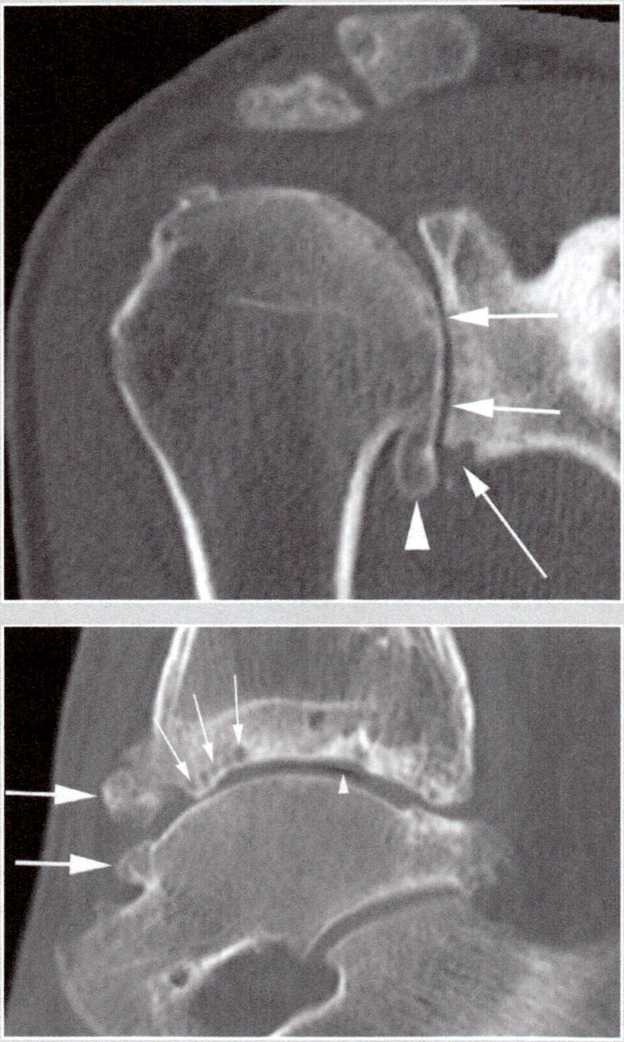

Figure 5.8 Use of computed tomography for evaluation of osteoarthritis. **A**, Coronal computed tomography (CT) image of the shoulder in advanced post-traumatic instability osteoarthritis. There is severe joint space narrowing (JSN) of the glenohumeral joint (short arrows). In addition, a large inferior humeral osteophyte is depicted (arrowhead) and a small subchondral cyst in the inferior glenoid is shown (long arrow). **B**, Sagittal CT image of post-traumatic ankle osteoarthritis. Large anterior osteophytes are depicted at the tibiotalar joint margin (large arrows). In addition, anterior JSN and small subchondral cysts are observed (small arrows). Note the intraarticular vacuum phenomenon, visualised as a hypodense intraarticular line, a common finding in osteoarthritic joints (see Figure 5.6). Figure courtesy of Drs D Hayashi, FW Roemer and A Guermazi.

Superior delineation of small focal cartilage defects by arthrography

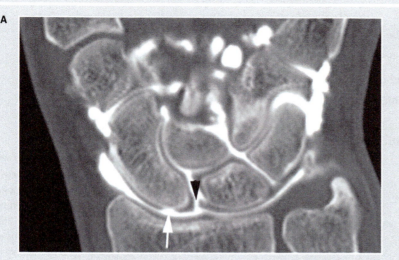

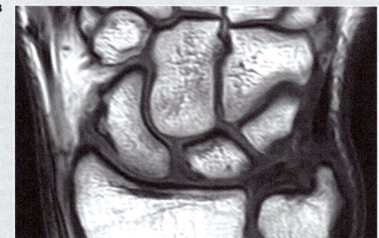

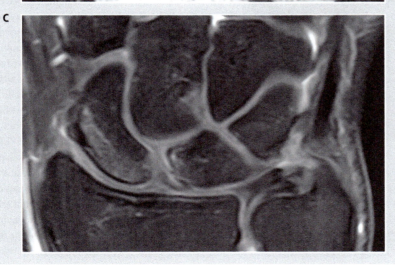

Figure 5.9 Superior delineation of small focal cartilage defects by arthrography.
A, Coronal computed tomography image of the wrist shows a focal full-thickness defect of the scaphoid at the radial articular surface (arrow). In addition, note the full thickness tear of the scapholunate ligament (arrowhead).
B, Corresponding T1-weighted nonarthrographic magnetic resonance imaging (MRI) shows a normal cartilaginous surface and ligament is inferiorly visualised.
C, Proton density-weighted MRI with fat suppression depicts subtle bone marrow oedema in the scaphoid but no articular surface damage of the scaphoid.
Figure courtesy of Drs D Hayashi, FW Roemer and A Guermazi.

Nuclear medicine

Positron emission tomography can be used to detect metabolic changes in target tissues. Increased uptake of 2-^{18}F-fluoro-2-deoxy–d-glucose can be seen in periarticular regions, inflamed synovium, the intercondylar notch and in areas of subchondral bone marrow corresponding to MRI-detected bone marrow lesions (Figure 5.10) [16,17].

2-^{18}F-fluoro-2-deoxy–D-glucose positron emission tomography

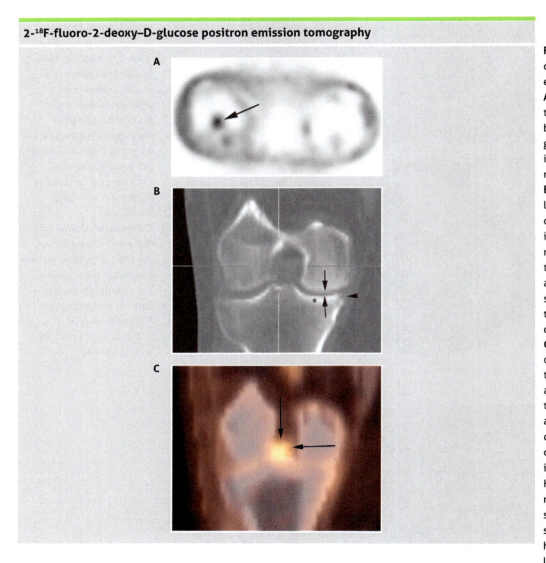

Figure 5.10 2-^{18}F-fluoro-2-deoxy–D-glucose positron emission tomography. **A**, Axial positron emission tomography (PET) image of both knees shows marked glucose uptake in the intercondylar notch of the right knee. **B**, Reconstructed low-resolution coronal computed tomography (CT) image depicts joint space narrowing of the medial tibiofemoral joint (arrows) and subchondral tibial sclerosis (*). In addition, there is a small medial tibial osteophyte (arrowhead). **C**, Coronal fusion image of PET and CT localises the pathologic glucose accumulation clearly to the intercondylar notch around the posterior cruciate ligament, the most common site of synovitis in knee osteoarthritis. Hypermetabolic findings represent peri-ligamentous synovitis. Note the high sensitivity of PET for hypermetabolism but the low specificity and poor spatial localisation without the support of additional cross-sectional imaging with CT or magnetic resonance imaging. Figure courtesy of Drs D Hayashi, FW Roemer and A Guermazi.

Summary of imaging findings in various osteoarthritis-affected joints

Osteoarthritis can affect various joints of the body, including the hand, shoulder, hip, knee, spine and sacroiliac joints. Typical imaging findings that affect these joints are summarised in Table 5.2. An illustration of multimodality imaging assessment with pathological correlation is presented in Figure 5.11 (see page 78), depicting end stage hip osteoarthritis using MRI and radiography as the primary assessment tools prior to total hip replacement.

Typical imaging findings of various osteoarthritis-affected joints

Joint	Imaging features

Hand	• JSN/loss, subchondral eburnation, marginal osteophyte formation, small ossicles in distal and proximal interphalangeal (DIP and PIP) joints
	  – Osteophytosis at DIP is called Heberden's nodes
	  – Osteophytosis at PIP is called Bouchard nodes
	• Radial subluxation of first metacarpal base
	• JSN and eburnation of trapezioscaphoid area

Shoulder	• Rotator cuff pathology • Labral tears • Osseous changes reflecting previous dislocation
Hip	• Acetabular and femoral osteophytes, sclerosis and subchondral cysts • Thickening/buttressing of medial femoral cortex • Superolateral subluxation of femoral head • Medial/axial subluxation with or without protrusio acetabuli • Signs of femoroacetabular impingement
Knee	• Medial tibiofemoral compartment is more commonly affected than lateral compartment • Tibiofemoral joint is more commonly affected than patellofemoral joint • Varus malalignment
Spine	• Sclerosis with narrowing of intervertebral apophyseal joints • Osteophytosis associated with disc pathology • Peridiscal endplate changes Modic type I–III • Spinal canal stenosis • Ligamentum flavum hypertrophy • Narrowing of neural foramina
Sacroiliac	• Can be bilateral or unilateral • If unilateral, the affected side is contralateral to the bad hip • Diffuse loss of joint space • Well-defined line of sclerosis, particularly on the iliac side of the joint • Bridging osteophytes at superior and inferior limits of joint

Table 5.2 Typical imaging findings of various osteoarthritis-affected joints. DIP, distal interphalangeal; JSN, joint space narrowing; PIP, proximal interphalangeal.

Multimodality imaging of severe hip osteoarthritis with pathologic correlation

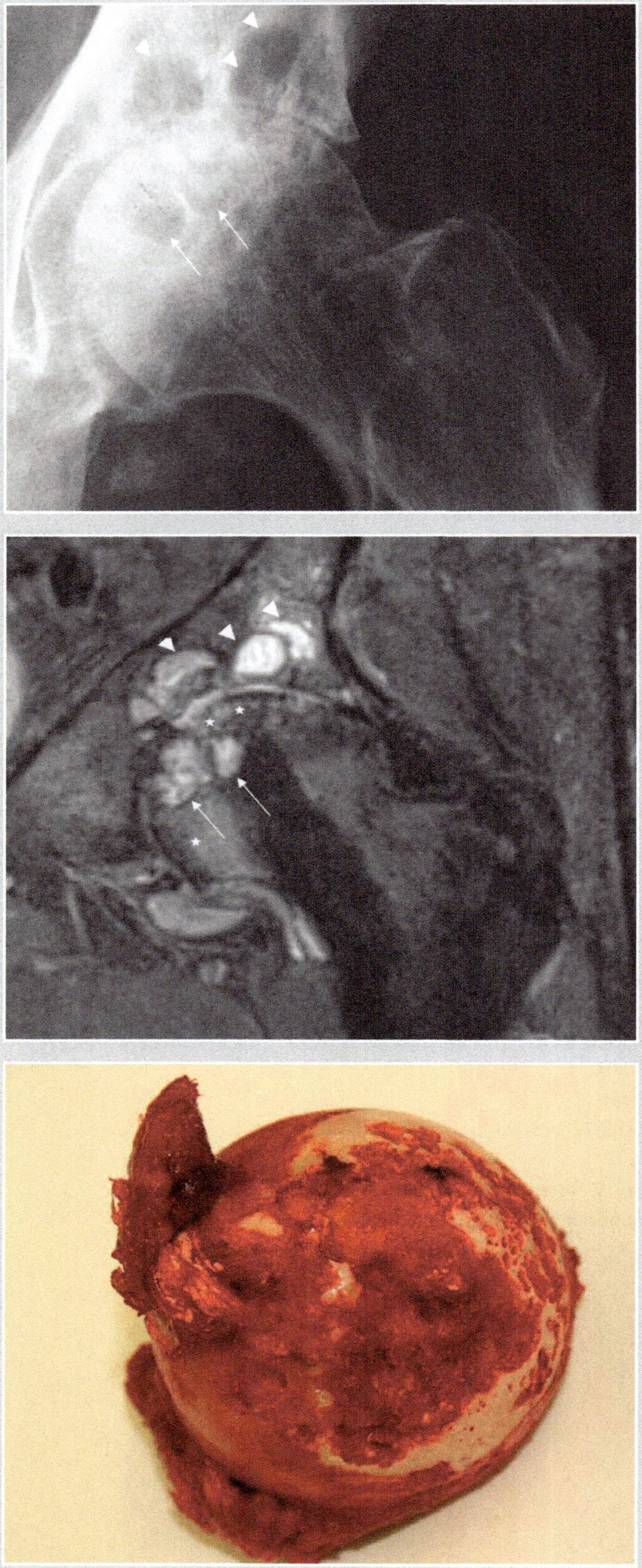

Figure 5.11 Multimodality imaging of severe hip osteoarthritis with pathologic correlation
A, Anteroposterior (AP) radiograph shows marked joint space narrowing and an acetabular osteophyte. There are also distinct subchondral cystic lesions in the femoral head (arrows) and acetabulum (arrowheads).
B, Coronal fat-suppressed proton density-weighted magnetic resonance imaging (MRI) depicts these subchondral cysts as hyperintense, fluid-equivalent lesions in the acetabulum (arrowheads) and femoral head (arrows). Note the marked diffuse bone marrow oedema visualised as areas of hyperintensity in the femoral head (*).
C, Macroscopic specimen shows diffuse cartilage loss of the articular surface of the femoral head (depicted on photograph as haemorrhagic areas). Subchondral changes cannot be visualised by surface photography.
(continues opposite).

Multimodality imaging of severe hip osteoarthritis with pathologic correlation *(continued)*

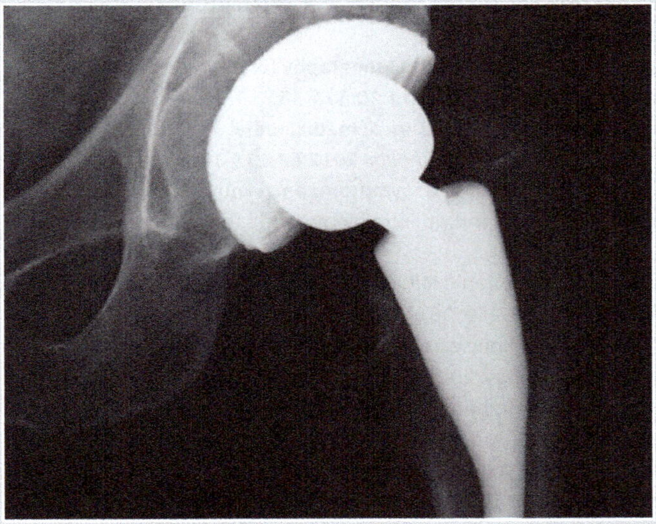

Figure 5.11 Multimodality imaging of severe hip osteoarthritis with pathologic correlation *(continued)*.
D, Macroscopic section through femoral head confirms MRI-depicted cystic lesions (arrows).
E, Haematoxylin-eosin stain of histologic specimen of the femoral head (corresponding to MRI B in this figure) confirms large subchondral cysts of the femoral head (arrows). Eosinophilic changes of the femoral head in the subchondral bone represent a mixture of oedema, subchondral sclerosis and fibrosis (asterisks).
F, Postsurgical AP radiograph of the same left hip after total joint replacement.
Figure courtesy of Drs D Hayashi, FW Roemer and A Guermazi.

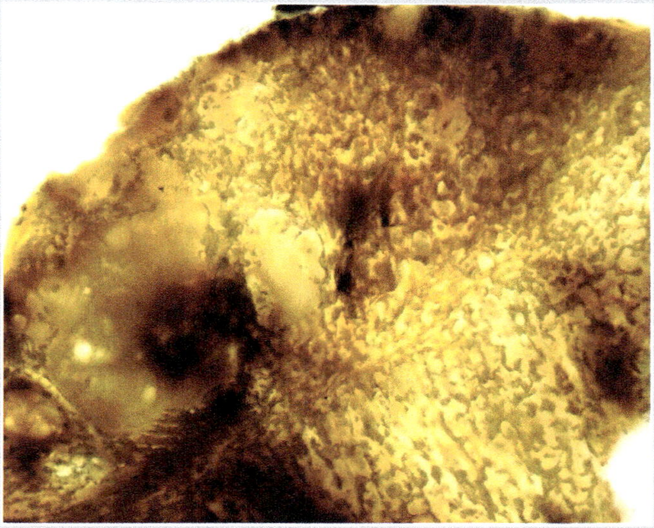

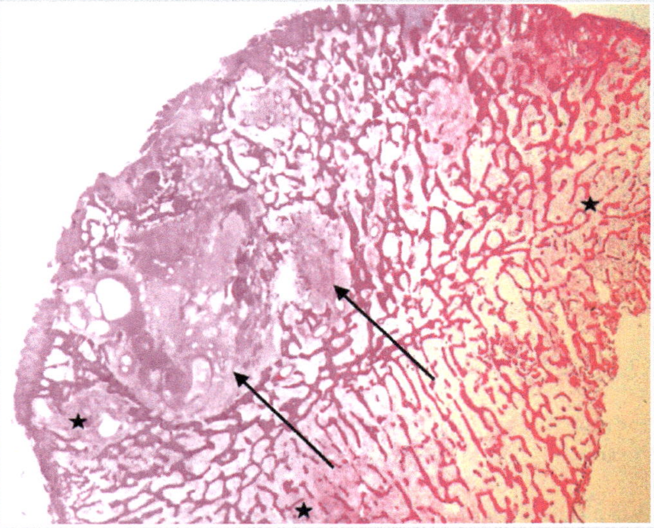

Future directions

Conventional radiography is still the first and most widely used imaging technique for evaluation of people with osteoarthritis. However, the ability of MRI to image the knee as a whole organ and to directly visualise lesions that are not detected with radiography is crucial to understanding the natural history of the disease, and ensures that MRI will play an important role in guiding future therapies. Ultrasound and contrast-enhanced MRI are particularly useful for imaging osteoarthritis-related synovitis.

References

1   Guermazi A, Hunter DJ, Roemer FW. Plain radiography and magnetic resonance imaging diagnostics in osteoarthritis: validated staging and scoring. *J Bone Joint Surg Am.* 2009;91(suppl 1):54-62.
2   Altman R, Asch E, Bloch D, et al. Development of criteria for the classification and reporting of osteoarthritis. Classification of osteoarthritis of the knee. Diagnostic and Therapeutic Criteria Committee of the American Rheumatism Association. *Arthritis Rheum.* 1986;29:1039-1049.
3   Kellgren JH, Lawrence JS. Radiological assessment of osteo-arthrosis. *Ann Rheum Dis.* 1957;16:494-502.
4   Altman RD, Gold GE. Atlas of individual radiographic features in osteoarthritis, revised. *Osteoarthritis Cartilage.* 2007;15(suppl A):A1-A56.
5   Peterfy CG, Gold G, Eckstein F, Cicuttini F, Dardzinski B, Stevens R. MRI protocols for whole-organ assessment of the knee in osteoarthritis. *Osteoarthritis Cartilage.* 2006;14(suppl A):A95-A111.
6   Roemer FW, Guermazi A. MR imaging-based semiquantitative assessment in osteoarthritis. *Radiol Clin North Am.* 2009;47:633-654.
7   Link TM. MR imaging in osteoarthritis: hardware, coils, and sequences. *Radiol Clin North Am.* 2009;47:617-632.
8   Hayashi D, Roemer FW, Katur A, et al. Imaging of synovitis in osteoarthritis: current status and outlook. *Semin Arthritis Rheum.* 2011;41:116-130.
9   Karim Z, Wakefield RJ, Quinn M, et al. Validation and reproducibility of ultrasonography in the detection of synovitis in the knee: a comparison with arthroscopy and clinical examination. *Arthritis Rheum.* 2004;50:387-394.
10 Walther M, Harms H, Krenn V, Radke S, Faehndrich T-P, Gohlke F. Correlation of power Doppler sonography with vascularity of the synovial tissue of the knee joint in patients with osteoarthritis and rheumatoid arthritis. *Arthritis Rheum.* 2001;44:331-338.
11 Saarakkala S, Waris P, Waris V, et al. Diagnostic performance of knee ultrasonography for detecting degenerative changes of articular cartilage. *Osteoarthritis Cartilage.* 2012;20:376-381.
12 Kawaguchi K, Enokida M, Otsuki R, Teshima R. Ultrasonographic evaluation of medial radial displacement of the medial meniscus in knee osteoarthritis. *Arthritis Rheum.* 2012;64:173-180.
13 Keen HI, Wakefield RJ, Hensor EMA, Emery P, Conaghan PG. Response of symptoms and synovitis to intra-muscular methylprednisolone in osteoarthritis of the hand: an ultrasonographic study. *Rheumatology (Oxford).* 2010;49:1093-1100.
14 Hechelhammer L, Pfirmann CWA, Zanetti M, Hodler J, Boos N, Schmid MR. Imaging findings predicting the outcome of cervical facet joint blocks. *Eur Radiol.* 2007;17:959-964.
15 Vande Berg BC, Lecouvet FE, Poilvache P, et al. Assessment of knee cartilage in cadavers with dual-detector spiral CT arthrography and MR imaging. *Radiology.* 2002;222:430-436.
16 Nakamura H, Masuko K, Yudoh K, et al. Positron emission tomography with ^{18}F-FDG in osteoarthritic knee. *Osteoarthritis Cartilage.* 2007;15:673-681.
17 Elzinga EH, van der Laken CJ, Comans EFI, Lammertsma AA, Dijkmans BAC, Voskuyl AE. 2-Deoxy-2-[F-18]fluoro-d-glucose joint uptake on positron emission tomography images: rheumatoid arthritis versus osteoarthritis. *Mol Imaging Biol.* 2007;9:357-360.

Chapter 6
Treatment of osteoarthritis

David Hunter

In the absence of a cure for osteoarthritis, current therapeutic modalities are primarily aimed at reducing pain and improving joint function by targeting symptom relief, without facilitating any improvement in the joint structure itself [1]. The management of osteoarthritis should be individualised so that it conforms to the specific findings of the clinical examination (Figure 6.1) [2]. This is especially the case for patients with obesity, malalignment and/or muscle weakness. Comprehensive management always includes a combination of treatment options that are directed towards the common goal of improving the patient's pain and tolerance for functional activity. Treatment plans should never be defined rigidly based on the X-ray appearance of the joint, but instead remain flexible so that they can be altered in line with the functional and symptomatic responses obtained [2]. Guidelines recommend that the hierarchy of management should consist of nonpharmacological modalities first, then drugs and then surgery [3–7].

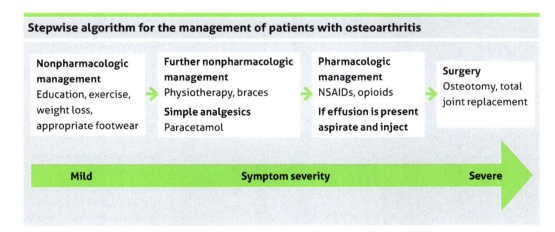

Figure 6.1 Stepwise algorithm for the management of patients with osteoarthritis. This is an example of a treatment algorithm that can be modified according to the patient's response and the clinician's preference. It highlights the encompassing need to consider nonpharmacological management as first-line treatment for all patients. NSAIDs, Nonsteroidal anti-inflammatory drugs. Data from Hunter & Felson [2]. © 2006, reproduced with permission from the British Medical Journal Publishing Group.

This publication has been made possible through an educational grant from SERVIER.

N. Arden et al., *Atlas of Osteoarthritis*, DOI 10.1007/978-1-910315-16-3_6,
© Springer Healthcare 2014

Nonpharmacological treatments

Self-management and education

All patients should be encouraged to participate in self-management programs (such as those conducted by the Arthritis Foundation [8]) that offer information on the natural history of osteoarthritis and provide resources for social support and instructions on coping skills [9,10].

The majority of individuals with arthritis are either overweight or obese [11]. There is good evidence for the efficacy of weight management [12], and this is advocated by most osteoarthritis guidelines [4–7]. However, in practice, weight management is not frequently implemented [13–15]. Another pivotal yet often ignored aspect of the conservative management of osteoarthritis is exercise. Although guidelines routinely advocate exercise [2–5,16,17], clinical practice does not reflect this recommendation [13–15].

Osteoarthritis and other obesity-related diseases and conditions place an enormous physical and financial burden on healthcare systems [18]. Weight loss has been universally recommended as a treatment for knee osteoarthritis [3–7], but is not always attainable due to patient and physician challenges in adhering to guidelines [14,19]. Recent data indicate that intensive dietary restriction plus exercise safely achieved a mean long-term (18 months) weight loss of 11.4% and yielded a 50% improvement in osteoarthritis symptoms (Figure 6.2) [20]. The wider adoption of dietary restrictions combined with exercise has a marked potential for reducing the burden of disability related to the increasing prevalence of osteoarthritis.

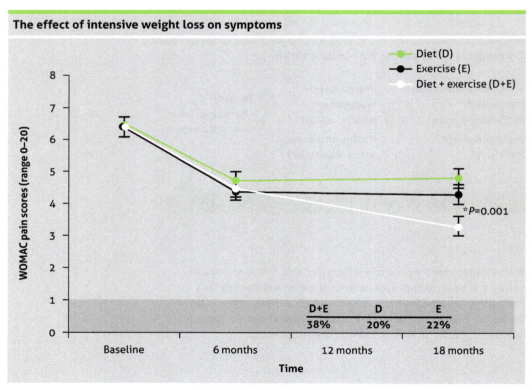

The effect of intensive weight loss on symptoms

Figure 6.2 The effect of intensive weight loss on symptoms. Mean (±SE) Western Ontario and McMaster Universities Osteoarthritis Index (WOMAC) pain scores (adjusted for gender, body mass index [BMI] and baseline values) across the 18-month intervention period. Baseline mean is overall for the three groups. Combined intensive dietary restriction and exercise led to a mean long-term weight loss of 11.4%, with 50% symptom improvement. At 18 months, 40% of participants in the diet plus exercise group reported little or no pain, with pain scores of 0 or 1 on a scale of 0–20, compared to around 20% of the diet-only and exercise-only groups. Data from Messier et al [20].

Exercise

Exercise is essential for all people with knee osteoarthritis, irrespective of disease severity age, comorbidity, pain severity or disability. Meta-analyses have found small-to-moderate effects in pain and function with exercise [21], similar to those achieved with analgesics and nonsteroidal anti-inflammatory drugs (NSAIDs).

High-intensity, home-based strength training can produce substantial improvements in strength, pain, physical function and quality of life in people with knee osteoarthritis (Figure 6.3) [22–28]. Given the deficits in muscle function present with knee osteoarthritis, muscle rehabilitation plays an important role in disease management in general and in reducing symptoms and improving function in particular. Table 6.1 lists the practical aspects of prescribing

The effect of quadriceps strengthening on physical function in knee osteoarthritis trials

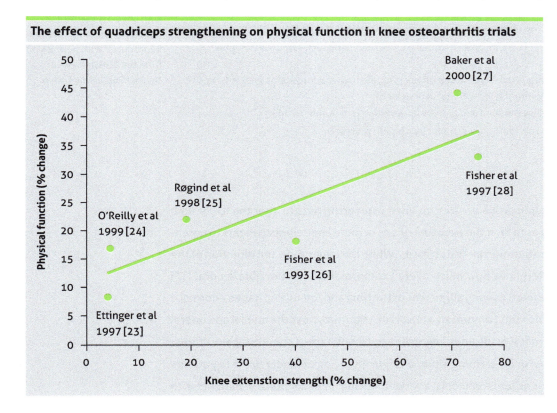

Figure 6.3 The effect of quadriceps strengthening on physical function in knee osteoarthritis trials. Improvements in knee extension strength are directly related to improvements in physical function. This figure shows the association between change in strength and change in physical function in published studies of exercise in knee osteoarthritis. Physical function is self-reported. r=0.877; *P*=0.02. Data from Baker et al [22]. Reproduced with permission from Dr K Baker and the *Journal of Rheumatology*.

Summary of exercise prescription for muscle rehabilitation

- Refer the patient to a health care professional for appropriate exercise prescription
- Supervised group or individual treatments are superior to independent home exercise for pain reduction
- Supplement home exercise with initial group exercise
- Exercise handouts or audiovisual material alone are ineffective
- Target quadriceps, hamstrings and hip abductors for strengthening
- Minimise compressive joint forces
- Clinical outcome is not influenced by the type of strengthening exercise
- Use a combined program of strengthening, flexibility and functional exercises
- Use strategies to maximise long-term patient compliance with exercise

Table 6.1 Summary of exercise prescription for muscle rehabilitation. Data from Bennell et al [29]. Reproduced with permission from Elsevier.

exercise for patients and reviews the current evidence on the optimum mode of delivery, type of exercise and dosage [29].

While exercise is a core treatment for knee osteoarthritis, adherence to exercise regimens is difficult to maintain, with research indicating that lack of adherence limits long-term effectiveness (Table 6.2) [30].

Strategies to facilitate long-term adherence to exercise and physical activity in people with knee osteoarthritis
Educate the patient about the disease and the benefits of exercise
Develop the exercise/physical activity plan with the patient and vary to maintain interest and enthusiasm
Use a graded progressive exercise/physical activity prescription and ensure pain/discomfort is not excessive during or after exercise
Initiate exercise under expert instruction and supervise exercise sessions if possible
Supplement face-to-face instruction with other materials; eg, written handouts, video/DVD/online demonstrations
Incorporate behavioural techniques to increase self efficacy; eg, positive reinforcement, goal setting, use of an exercise contract, self-monitoring via diary, pedometer
Include spouse/family in exercise program and garner support from family and friends
Monitor over the long-term via periodic reassessment by a health professional

Table 6.2 Strategies to facilitate long-term adherence to exercise and physical activity in people with knee osteoarthritis. Data from Bennell et al [30]. Reproduced with permission from the British Medical Journal Publishing Group.

Assistive devices

The shared goal of many noninvasive devices for knee osteoarthritis is to alter the lower limb biomechanics in such a way as to limit the exposure of one or more knee compartments to potentially damaging and provocative mechanical stresses. While the magnitude and direction of the ground reaction forces determines how much overall compressive load the tibiofemoral (TF) joint routinely sustains, the relative bony alignment of the tibia and femur also has an enormous impact on the manner in which this compressive load is distributed across the medial and lateral compartments. Improved frontal plane knee alignment and mediolateral stability against thrust are commonly cited reasons for prescribing either a valgus-inducing unloader brace to patients with medial TF osteoarthritis or, less commonly, a varus-inducing unloader brace to patients with lateral TF osteoarthritis (Figure 6.4) [31,32].

Use of brace device for symptomatic knee osteoarthritis

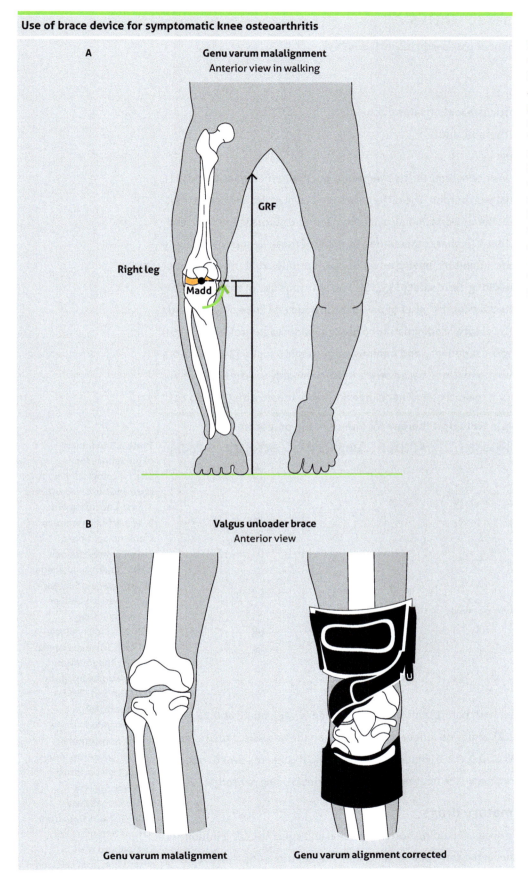

A

Genu varum malalignment
Anterior view in walking

GRF

Right leg

Madd

B

Valgus unloader brace
Anterior view

Genu varum malalignment

Genu varum alignment corrected

Figure 6.4 Use of brace device for symptomatic knee osteoarthritis. **A**, Loading of the knee with genu varum, or bowlegged, malalignment. Genu varum increases the adduction moment (Madd) at the knee and the magnitude of compressive load on the medial TF compartment. **B**, Correction of genu varum malalignment using a valgus unloader brace. Data from Gross [32]. © 2010, reproduced with permission from Elsevier.

Pharmacological treatments

The pharmacological management of osteoarthritis includes [33]:

- Simple analgesics;
- NSAIDs;
- Intra-articular therapies (corticosteroids, hyaluronic acid);
- Supplements or alternative therapy; and
- Disease modification therapy.

Current drug treatment options reduce osteoarthritis symptoms, but their efficacy is limited [21], leaving patients with a substantial pain burden. The difference between placebo and active treatment for many widely used current therapies, including hyaluronic acid and glucosamine, is exceedingly difficult to detect [34,35]. This is further compounded by many of these agents, particularly cyclooxygenase-2 (COX-2) specific inhibitors, having adverse-event profiles that raise a number of legitimate concerns about their long-term safety [35,36]. The judicious use of topical NSAIDs has been demonstrated to be effective for the relief of pain in both hand and knee osteoarthritis compared with placebo [37,38]. This route of administration possibly reduces gastrointestinal (GI) adverse reactions by maximising local delivery and minimising systemic toxicity [39]. Table 6.3 provides an overview of the recommendations, based on the most commonly used guidelines, for different pharmacological agents in the management of knee and hip osteoarthritis [3–7,40,41].

Summary of guidelines for pharmacological therapy for knee and hip osteoarthritis

Agent/drug class	AAOS [6]	ACR [7]	EULAR [3,4]	NICE [40]	OARSI [5]
Acetaminophen	1	1	1	1	1
COX-2 specific inhibitors	2	2	2	2	1
Tramadol		2			
Opiates		2	2	2	2
NSAIDs	1	1	2	2	1
Topical NSAIDs	2	2	1	1	1
Capsaicin		2	1	2	1
Topical salicylate		2	1	NR	
Intra-articular steroids	Short term only	1	2	2	2
Intra-articular hyaluronic acid	NR	2	2	NR	2
Glucosamine and chondroitin	NR		2	NR	2

Table 6.3 Summary of guidelines for pharmacological therapy for knee and hip osteoarthritis. 1, First-line treatment; 2, second-line treatment; blank, no opinion in the recommendations; AAOS, American Academy of Orthopaedic Surgeons; ACR, American College of Rheumatology; COX-2, cyclooxygenase-2; EULAR, European League Against Rheumatism; NICE, National Institute of Health and Clinical Excellence; NR, not recommended for use; NSAID, nonsteroidal anti-inflammatory drugs; OARSI, Osteoarthritis Research Society International. Data from [3–7,40]. Data from Harvey & Hunter [41]. Reproduced with permission from Elsevier.

Simple analgesics

The effect size (ES) for pain relief with paracetamol/acetaminophen is very small, at 0.14 (95% confidence interval [CI]: 0.05, 0.22), and is no longer significant when the analysis is restricted to high-quality trials (ES=0.10, 95% CI: 0.0, 0.23) (Figure 6.5). In the light of concerns over GI toxicity, the role of paracetamol/acetaminophen in the treatment of osteoarthritis is being revised [5,42–47].

Nonsteroidal anti-inflammatory drugs

Nonsteroidal anti-inflammatory drugs, including both traditional and specific COX-2 inhibitors, provide significant health benefits in the treatment of pain and inflammation [46]. However, they

Pain relief effect of paracetamol

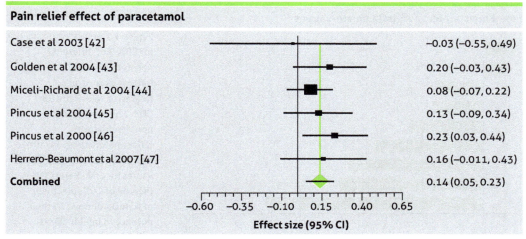

Case et al 2003 [42]	−0.03 (−0.55, 0.49)
Golden et al 2004 [43]	0.20 (−0.03, 0.43)
Miceli-Richard et al 2004 [44]	0.08 (−0.07, 0.22)
Pincus et al 2004 [45]	0.13 (−0.09, 0.34)
Pincus et al 2000 [46]	0.23 (0.03, 0.44)
Herrero-Beaumont et al 2007 [47]	0.16 (−0.011, 0.43)
Combined	0.14 (0.05, 0.23)

Effect size (95% CI): −0.60 −0.35 −0.10 0.15 0.40 0.65

Figure 6.5 Pain relief effect of paracetamol. CI, confidence interval. Data from [42–47]. Data from Zhang et al [5]. Reproduced with permission from Elsevier.

are associated with an increased risk of serious GI [48] and cardiovascular adverse events [49]. Both beneficial and adverse effects are due to the same mechanism of action—the inhibition of COX-dependent prostanoids (Figures 6.6–6.9, Table 6.4; see pages 87–90) [50–53].

COX-1 versus COX-2

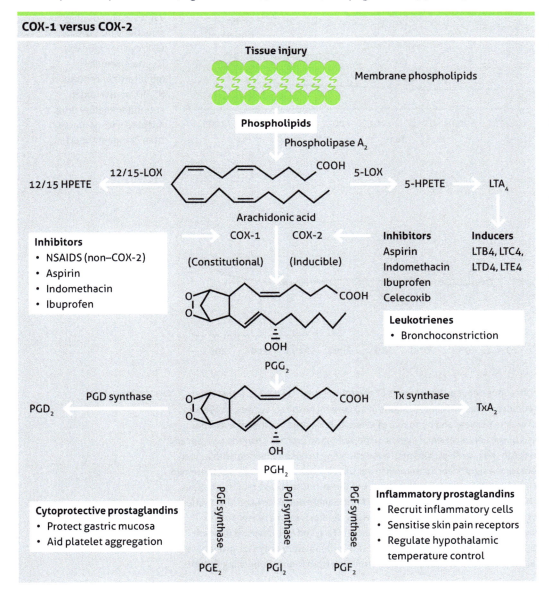

Figure 6.6 COX-1 versus COX-2. Representative biosynthetic pathway of prostaglandin (PG) biosynthesis from arachidonic acid (AA) via cyclooxygenase (COX)-1/COX-2 isoform catalysis. The NSAIDs, aspirin, indomethacin and ibuprofen, are nonselective inhibitors of COX isozymes, whereas celecoxib exhibits selective COX-2 inhibition. LOX, lipoxygenase; LT, leukotriene. Adapted with permission from Rao & Knaus [50].

Selectivity for COX-2 of different nonsteroidal anti-inflammatory drugs

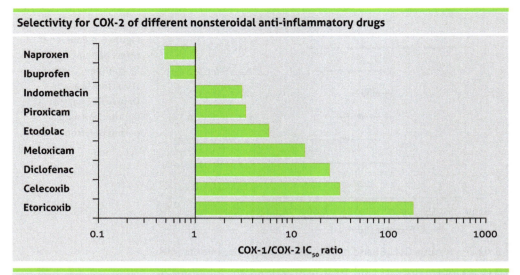

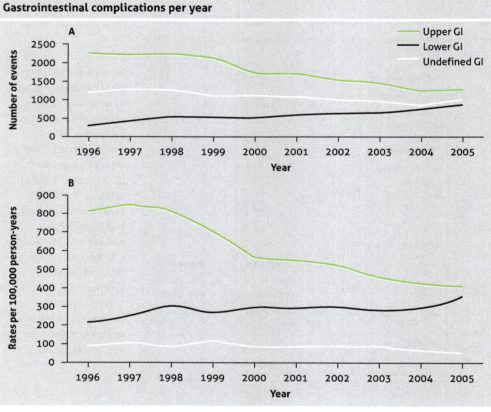

Figure 6.7 Selectivity for COX-2 of different nonsteroidal anti-inflammatory drugs. Degree of selectivity for COX-2 by the different nonsteroidal anti-inflammatory drugs in vitro, expressed as ratio of IC_{50} values for COX-1 and COX-2 (degree of COX selectivity of NSAIDs, defined by their potency to inhibit COX-1 and COX-2 activities in vitro by 50%). Higher values of COX-1/COX-2 IC_{50} ratio (>1) mirror higher selectivity versus COX-2; lower values (<1) mirror higher selectivity for COX-1. COX, cyclooxygenase; IC_{50}, half maximal inhibitory concentration; NSAID, nonsteroidal anti-inflammatory drug. Adapted with permission from Patrignani et al [51].

Figure 6.8 Gastrointestinal complications per year. Time trends of gastrointestinal (GI) events. Data is from a study of hospitalised patients admitted due to GI complications in 10 general hospitals between 1996 and 2005 in Spain. **A**, Total number of events per year and by source of event. **B**, Estimated number of event per 100,000 person-years on the basis of the adjudication of events in the validation process. Over the past decade, there has been a progressive change in the overall picture of GI events leading to hospitalisation, with a clear decreasing trend in upper GI events and a significant increase in lower GI events, causing the rates of these two GI complications to converge. Overall, mortality has also decreased, but the in-hospital case fatality of upper or lower GI complication events has remained constant. The reasons for the sharp decrease in hospitalisations because of upper GI events is not well defined, but on the basis of earlier reports it seems reasonable to accept that a decrease in *Helicobacter pylori* infection, a probable cohort effect, and a progressive increase in implementing prevention strategies in patients taking nonsteroidal anti-inflammatory drugs are probably the key players. Data from Lanas et al [52]. © 2009, reproduced with permission from Nature Publishing Group.

Morbidity rate ratios for nonsteroidal anti-inflammatories compared with placebo

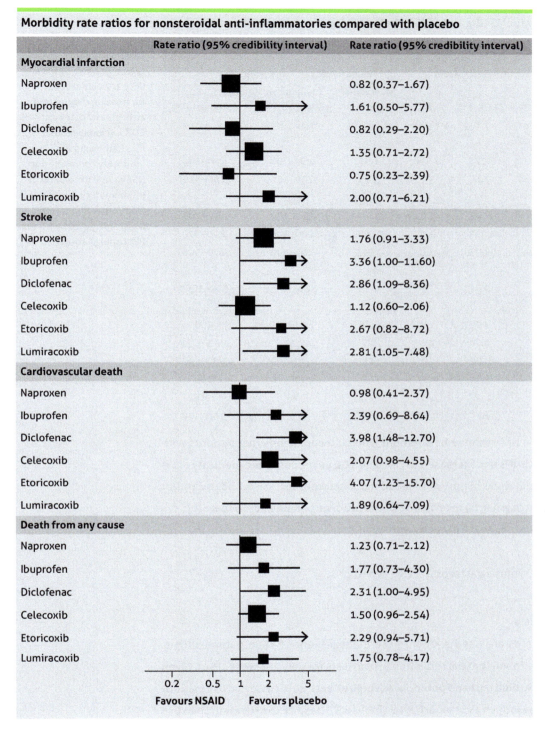

	Rate ratio (95% credibility interval)	Rate ratio (95% credibility interval)
Myocardial infarction		
Naproxen		0.82 (0.37–1.67)
Ibuprofen		1.61 (0.50–5.77)
Diclofenac		0.82 (0.29–2.20)
Celecoxib		1.35 (0.71–2.72)
Etoricoxib		0.75 (0.23–2.39)
Lumiracoxib		2.00 (0.71–6.21)
Stroke		
Naproxen		1.76 (0.91–3.33)
Ibuprofen		3.36 (1.00–11.60)
Diclofenac		2.86 (1.09–8.36)
Celecoxib		1.12 (0.60–2.06)
Etoricoxib		2.67 (0.82–8.72)
Lumiracoxib		2.81 (1.05–7.48)
Cardiovascular death		
Naproxen		0.98 (0.41–2.37)
Ibuprofen		2.39 (0.69–8.64)
Diclofenac		3.98 (1.48–12.70)
Celecoxib		2.07 (0.98–4.55)
Etoricoxib		4.07 (1.23–15.70)
Lumiracoxib		1.89 (0.64–7.09)
Death from any cause		
Naproxen		1.23 (0.71–2.12)
Ibuprofen		1.77 (0.73–4.30)
Diclofenac		2.31 (1.00–4.95)
Celecoxib		1.50 (0.96–2.54)
Etoricoxib		2.29 (0.94–5.71)
Lumiracoxib		1.75 (0.78–4.17)

0.2　0.5　1　2　5

Favours NSAID　　**Favours placebo**

Figure 6.9 Morbidity rate ratios for nonsteroidal anti-inflammatories compared with placebo. Although uncertainty remains, little evidence exists to suggest that any of the nonsteroidal anti-inflammatory drugs (NSAIDs) are safe in terms of cardiovascular events. Naproxen appears to be the least harmful. Cardiovascular risk needs to be taken into account when prescribing any NSAID. Data from Trelle et al [53]. © 2011, reproduced with permission from the British Medical Journal Publishing Group.

Inhibition data, selectivity for NSAIDs and COX-1/2 clinical dose for treating rheumatoid arthritis and osteoarthritis

Drug	Trade name	Whole blood assay IC$_{50}$ (µM)		Selectivity index	Clinical dose	
		COX-1	COX-2		Rheumatoid arthritis	Osteoarthritis
Aspirin	Aspirin® Ecotrin®	1.7	>100	0.017	2600–3900	–
Diclofenac	Voltaren®	0.075	0.038	1.97	150–200	150–200
Ibuprofen	Advil® Motren®	7.6	7.2	1.05	1200–3200	1200–3200
Indomethacin	Indocin®	0.013	1.0	0.013	150–200	150–200
Ketoprofen	Orudis®	0.047	2.9	0.016	200–300	200–300
Fluorbiprofen	Fluorbiprofen® Ansaid®	0.075	5.5	0.013	200–300	200–300
Naproxen	Naprosyn® Aleve®	9.3	28	0.33	500–1000	500–1000
Nimesulide	Mesulid®	10	1.9	5.26	–	200
Meloxicam	Mobic®	5.7	2.1	2.7	7.5–15	7.5–15
Paracetamol	Tylenol®	>100	49	>2.04	2600–4000	2600–4000
Celecoxib	Celebrex®	6.7	0.87	7.7	200–400	200
Etoricoxib	Arcoxia®	116	1.1	105.4	90	60
Lumiracoxib	Prexige®	67	0.13	515	–	200–400

Table 6.4 Inhibition data, selectivity for NSAIDs and COX-1/2 clinical dose for treating rheumatoid arthritis and osteoarthritis. COX, cyclooxygenase; IC$_{50}$, half maximal inhibitory concentration; NSAID, nonsteroidal anti-inflammatory drug. Data from Rao & Knaus [50]. Rights managed by Nature Publishing Group.

The American Academy of Orthopaedic Surgeons (AAOS) recommends that patients with symptomatic knee osteoarthritis and increased GI risk (age ≥60 years, comorbid medical conditions, history of peptic ulcer disease, history of GI bleeding, concurrent corticosteroid use and/or the concomitant use of anticoagulants) receive one of the following analgesics for pain [6]:

- Paracetamol/acetaminophen (not to exceed 4 g/day);
- Topical NSAIDs;
- Nonselective oral NSAIDs plus a gastroprotective agent; or
- COX-2 specific inhibitors.

Intra-articular therapies

Intra-articular corticosteroids are used widely in the management of knee osteoarthritis. However, a Cochrane review found that the reduction in pain lasts for only 1–2 weeks [54]. Given this short duration of benefit, high cost and potential adverse effects, corticosteroid use may not be merited in a chronic disease such as osteoarthritis (Table 6.5). Despite the temptation to use these agents in patients with the features of clinical inflammation (such as a large effusion), the evidence to support this is limited.

The use of intra-articular injections of viscosupplements (eg, hyaluronic acid), usually given weekly for 3–5 weeks, has been extensively researched, but a recent meta-analysis found that the trials are generally of low quality and that viscosupplementation is associated with a small and clinically irrelevant reduction in pain but an increased risk of serious adverse events [55].

Overview of intra-articular steroids

Agent	Relative anti-inflammatory potency	Solubility	Dose
Hydrocortisone acetate	1	High	10–25 mg
Methylprednisolone acetate	5	Medium	20–80 mg
Triamcinolone acetonide	5	Medium	10–40 mg
Triamcinolone hexacetonide			10–20 mg
Betamethasone sodium phosphate and acetate	20	Low	0.25–2 mL

Table 6.5 Overview of intra-articular steroids. Injectable corticosteroids can be classified in terms of solubility and duration of action. High-solubility preparations have a short duration of action and low-solubility compounds have a long duration. This table shows the relative anti-inflammatory potencies of various injectable corticosteroids, with hydrocortisone used as the standard with a value of 1.0.

Antidepressants

Because some people with knee osteoarthritis also have depression and symptoms of neuropathic pain (shooting or burning pain, pins and needles), the role of centrally active agents, including selective serotonin and noradrenaline (norepinephrine) reuptake inhibitors, has been investigated. In a randomised controlled trial (RCT) of duloxetine versus placebo, 65% of participants in the duloxetine group reported a reduction in pain of more than 30%, compared with just 44% in the placebo group [56]. This was the result of a primary analgesic effect and not an elevation in mood or changes in anxiety or depression [38]. These agents may be useful in subgroups of patients with knee osteoarthritis.

Supplements or alternative therapy

The most commonly used alternative treatment is glucosamine. In clinical trials, glucosamine has a similar effect on pain to that of placebo, with industry-independent trials showing smaller effects than commercially funded ones [21] and most published studies show controversial effects on structure modification [57]. In contrast, a meta-analysis consisting of just three RCTs of two years' duration found that chondroitin had a small effect on symptoms and structure (ES 0.23) [58]. Both Vitamin D and fish oil are promising areas of current investigation.

Disease modification therapy

Once a popular area for drug development, with a multitude of discovery and preclinical programs at major pharmaceutical and biotech companies and dozens of compounds moving through pharmaceutical pipelines toward pivotal clinical trials, research on slowing or stopping the progression of cartilage loss and other structural changes in the joint has been significantly scaled back. This is due in large part to challenges over target identification and clinical development (Table 6.6, Figure 6.10; see pages 92-93) [59,60]. The cited references provide a detailed review of this complicated area including the lessons learned from prior disease-modifying osteoarthritis drug trials and the challenges that lie therein in trial conduct.

Pharmacologic agents currently in development for the treatment of osteoarthritis

Compound/product	Company	Primary indication	Stage of development	Mechanism of action (route)
Tanezumab	Pfizer	Pain	Phase III, trial halted due to FDA concerns with safety	Anti-NGF Ab (IV)
Fulranumab	Johnson & Johnson	Pain	Phase II, on clinical hold	Anti-NGF Ab (SC)
REGN475	Sanofi/Regeneron	Pain	Phase II, on clinical hold	Anti-NGF Ab (IV)
MEDI-578	Astra Zeneca	Pain	Phase I, on clinical hold	Anti-NGF Ab (IV)
PG110	Abbot	Pain	Phase I	Anti-NGF Ab (IV)
PF-04191834	Pfizer	Pain	Phase II, on clinical hold	5-LOX inhibitor (oral)
NSAID reformulation/ dose changes	multiple	Pain	Phase II/III	Prostaglandin inhibition; anti-inflammatory
HA reformulation/ dose change	Anika, Ferring, Seikagaku, Q-Med	Pain	Most Phase III or at FDA post-Phase III	Synovial fluid HA replacement (IA)
Hydros/Hydros TA	Carbylan Biosurgery	Pain	Phase II excluding US; July 2011 results announced superior pain relief and improved function	HA + steroid combination (IA)
BMP-7 (OP-1)	Stryker	Structure modification	Phase I/II	Pro-anabolic growth factor (IA)
Salmon calcitonin	Novartis	Structure modification	Phase III	Bone and articular surface contour preservation (oral)
PH-797804	Pfizer	Structure modification	Phase II	MAP kinase inhibitor
SD-6010	Pfizer	Structure modification	Phase II; joint space narrowing over 24 months	iNOS inhibitor
FGF-18	Merck-Serono	Structure modification	Phase I; change in cartilage thickness by MRI	Pro-anabolic growth factor (IA)
Autologous bone marrow stem cells	International Stemcell Services and others	Structure modification	Phase I/II; pain and cartilage mapping by MRI	Regenerative, pro-anabolic, anti-inflammatory
Canakinumab	Novartis	Structure modification	Phase II	Anti-IL-1 Ab (IA)
SAR-113945	Sanofi	Unknown	Phase I	IKK-beta kinase inhibitor (IA)
ABT-652	Abbott	Unknown	Phase II	Unknown
ASU	Laboratoires Expanscience	Structure modification	Phase III	Stimulates matrix synthesis and inhibitor of inflammation
Vitamin D3	National Institute of Arthritis and Musculoskeletal and Skin Diseases, University of Zurich	Structure modification	Phase II	Acts on vitamin D receptors in bone and cartilage
Collagen hydrolysate	Gelita	Structure modification	Phase II	Affects type 2 collagen turnover

Table 6.6 Pharmacologic agents currently in development for the treatment of osteoarthritis. Currently, clinical research efforts have dropped to only a small number of candidates still in later-stage trials. Most notably, these include intra-articular (IA) administration of the pro-anabolic agents osteogenic protein-1 (OP-1) and fibroblast growth factor-18 (FGF-18), in addition to an anti-catabolic inducible nitric oxide synthase (iNOS) inhibitor. The results of recently completed clinical trials evaluating oral salmon calcitonin are pending. There are also trials ongoing or being planned which evaluate cell therapy (eg, autologous mesenchymal stem cells) for structure modification effects. Ab, Antibody; ASU, avocado–soybean unsaponifiable; BMP, bone morphogenetic protein; FGF, fibroblast growth factor; HA, hyaloronic acid; IA, intra-articular; iNOS, inducible nitric oxide synthase; IV, intravenous; LOX, lipoxygenase; NGF, nerve growth factor; NSAID, nonsteroidal anti-inflamatory drug; SC, subcutaneous. Publicly available details of these trials can be found at www.clinicaltrials.gov. Data from Matthews & Hunter [59] and Hunter [60].

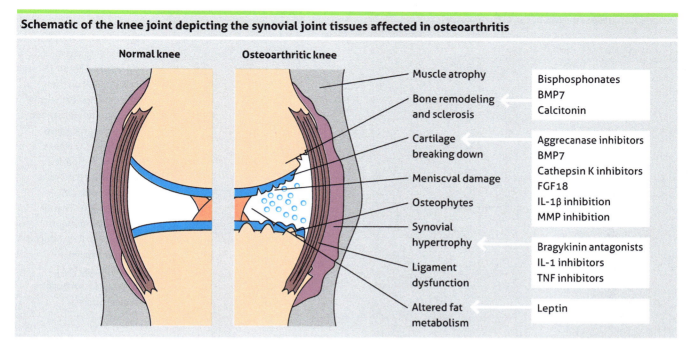

Schematic of the knee joint depicting the synovial joint tissues affected in osteoarthritis

Figure 6.10 Schematic of the knee joint depicting the synovial joint tissues affected in osteoarthritis. Consistent with the theory that osteoarthritis is a disease of the whole synovial joint, current disease-modifying osteoarthritis drug development is now targeting synovial-joint tissue structures, including bone, cartilage and synovium. Some of the agents that target these relevant tissues are listed here. BMP, bone morphogenetic protein; FGF, fibroblast growth factor; IL, interleukin; MMP, matrix metalloproteinase; TNF, tumour necrosis factor. Adapted from Hunter [60]. © 2010, rights managed by Nature Publishing Group.

Surgical treatments

Surgery should be considered only when symptoms can be managed by other treatment modalities [61].

Arthroscopy

The AAOS recommends that arthroscopic lavage or debridement (or both) and meniscal resection be performed only in patients with mechanical symptoms, such as the sudden onset of the inability to fully extend the knee or disabling, repeated catching or locking of the joint [6]. Arthroscopic debridement and meniscal resection remains the most frequently performed procedure by orthopaedic surgeons in most developed countries [62,63], with up to 1 million knee arthroscopies performed annually in the US alone (Figures 6.11 and 6.12; see page 94-95) [64]. This operation has no demonstrable effect on pain in knee osteoarthritis compared with more conservative modes of care [21,64,65].

Osteotomy

A recent systematic review of valgus high tibial osteotomy suggested that this intervention leads to improvements in pain and function [66]. Recovery is typically prolonged, but osteotomy may delay the need for total joint replacement for 5–10 years [67]. Currently, there is a debate as to the relative merits of osteotomy versus unicompartmental knee replacement, which warrants

Knee-pain assessments after arthroscopy

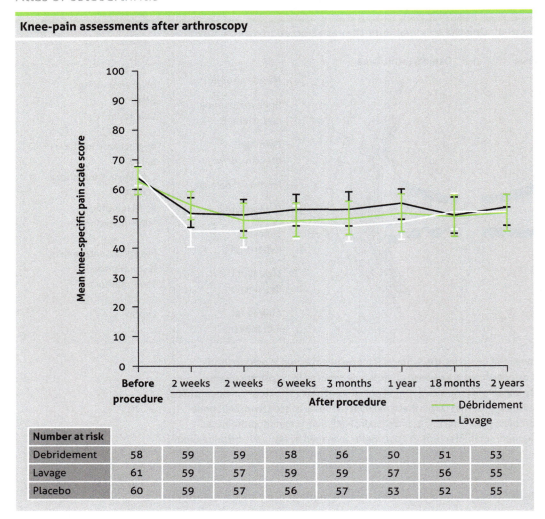

Number at risk

Debridement	58	59	59	58	56	50	51	53
Lavage	61	59	57	59	59	57	56	55
Placebo	60	59	57	56	57	53	52	55

Figure 6.11 Knee-pain assessments after arthroscopy. Mean values (and 95% CI) on the Knee-Specific Pain Scale. Assessments were made before the procedure and 2 weeks, 6 weeks, 3 months, 6 months, 12 months, 18 months and 24 months after the procedure. Higher scores indicate more severe pain. Reproduced with permission from Moseley [64]. © 2002, Massachusetts Medical Society.

further investigation in well-designed clinical trials [68]. It is important to note that no trials to date have compared osteotomy with conservative treatment.

Joint replacement

Joint arthroplasty is reserved for patients with severe disease (Figure 6.13) [66], defined as persistent moderate-to-severe pain, functional limitation and reduced quality of life despite optimal conservative treatment, combined with radiologic findings [69]. Patients should be referred to an orthopaedic surgeon when joint replacement is required, preferably before substantive functional decline has occurred as this may not be regained following surgery [70].

Arthroscopic procedure

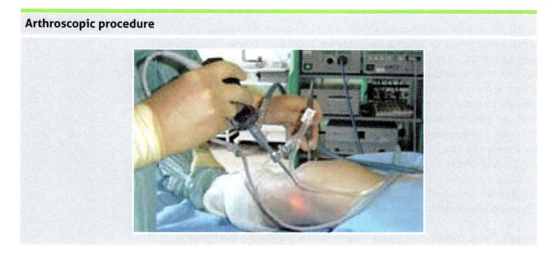

Figure 6.12 Arthroscopic procedure. Image courtesy of Dr D Hunter.

Bilateral total knee arthroplasties

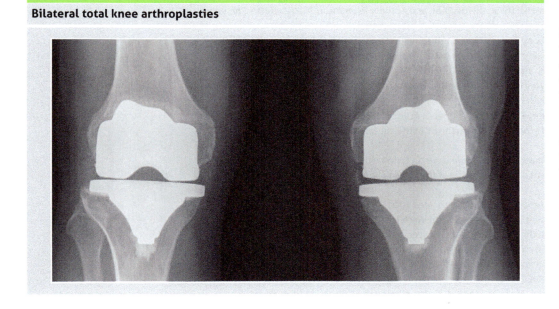

Figure 6.13 Bilateral total knee arthroplasties. Arthroplasty is an extremely cost-effective treatment for end-stage knee osteoarthritis. It is noted for high durability and excellent long-term survival. Image from Richmond [61]. © 2008, reproduced with permission from Elsevier.

References

1 Hunter DJ, Lo GH. The management of osteoarthritis: an overview and call to appropriate conservative treatment. *Rheum Dis Clin North Am.* 2008;34:689-712.
2 Hunter DJ, Felson DT. Osteoarthritis. *BMJ.* 2006;332:639-642.
3 Jordan KM, Arden NK, Doherty M, et al; Standing Committee for International Clinical Studies Including Therapeutic Trials. EULAR recommendations 2003: an evidence based approach to the management of knee osteoarthritis: report of a task force of the Standing Committee for International Clinical Studies Including Therapeutic Trials (ESCISIT). *Ann Rheum Dis.* 2003;62:1145-1155.
4 Zhang W, Doherty M, Arden N, et al; EULAR Standing Committee for International Clinical Studies Including Therapeutics. EULAR evidence based recommendations for the management of hip osteoarthritis: report of a task force of the EULAR Standing Committee for International Clinical Studies Including Therapeutics (ESCISIT). *Ann Rheum Dis.* 2005;64:669-681.
5 Zhang W, Moskowitz RW, Nuki G, et al. OARSI recommendations for the management of hip and knee osteoarthritis, Part II: OARSI evidence-based, expert consensus guidelines. *Osteoarthritis Cartilage.* 2008;16:137-162.

6   Richmond J, Hunter D, Irrgang JJ, Jet al; American Academy of Orthopaedic Surgeons Workgroup. Treatment of osteoarthritis of the knee (nonarthroplasty): full guideline. Rosemont, IL: American Academy of Orthopaedic Surgeons; 2008.

7   Hochberg MC, Altman RD, April KT, et al. American College of Rheumatology 2012 recommendations for the use of nonpharmacologic and pharmacologic therapies in osteoarthritis of the hand, hip, and knee. *Arthritis Care Res (Hoboken)*. 2012;64:465-474.

8   Superio-Cabuslay E, Ward MM, Lorig KR. Patient education interventions in osteoarthritis and rheumatoid arthritis: a meta-analytic comparison with nonsteroidal antiinflammatory drug treatment. *Arthritis Care Res*. 1996;9:292-301.

9   Arthritis Foundation website. Disease Center. Available at: www.arthritis.org/disease-center.php Accessed 8 October 2012.

10   Marks R, Allegrante JP, Lorig K. A review and synthesis of research evidence for self-efficacy-enhancing interventions for reducing chronic disability: implications for health education practice (part I). *Health Promot Pract*. 2005;6:37-43.

11   Felson DT, Lawrence RC, Dieppe PA, et al. Osteoarthritis: new insights. Part 1: the disease and its risk factors. *Ann Intern Med*. 2000;133:635-646.

12   Messier SP, Loeser RF, Miller GD, et al. Exercise and dietary weight loss in overweight and obese older adults with knee osteoarthritis: the Arthritis, Diet, and Activity Promotion Trial. *Arthritis Rheum*. 2004;50:1501-1510.

13   Hutchings A, Calloway M, Choy E, et al. The Longitudinal Examination of Arthritis Pain (LEAP) study: relationships between weekly fluctuations in patient-rated joint pain and other health outcomes. *J Rheumatol*. 2007;34:2291-2300.

14   DeHaan MN, Guzman J, Bayley MT, Bell MJ. Knee osteoarthritis clinical practice guidelines – how are we doing? *J Rheumatol*. 2007;34:2099-2105.

15   Jordan KM, Sawyer S, Coakley P, Smith HE, Cooper C, Arden NK. The use of conventional and complementary treatments for knee osteoarthritis in the community. *Rheumatology (Oxford)*. 2004;43:381-384.

16   American College of Rheumatology Subcommittee on Osteoarthritis Guidelines. Recommendations for the medical management of osteoarthritis of the hip and knee: 2000 update. *Arthritis Rheum*. 2000;43:1905-1915.

17   Hunter DJ. In the clinic. Osteoarthritis. *Ann Intern Med* 2007;147:ITC8-1-ITC8-16.

18   Wang YC, McPherson K, Marsh T, Gortmaker SL, Brown M. Health and economic burden of the projected obesity trends in the USA and the UK. *Lancet*. 2011;378:815-825.

19   Glazier RH, Dalby DM, Badley EM, et al. Management of common musculoskeletal problems: a survey of Ontario primary care physicians. *CMAJ*. 1998;158:1037-1040.

20   Messier S, Nicklas B, Legault C, et al. The Intensive Diet and Exercise for Arthritis (IDEA) trial: 18-month clinical outcomes. Paper presented at: 2011 American College of Rheumatology/Association of Rheumatology Health Professionals Annual Meeting; November 5–9, 2011; Chicago, IL.

21   Zhang W, Nuki G, Moskowitz RW, et al. OARSI recommendations for the management of hip and knee osteoarthritis: part III: changes in evidence following systematic cumulative update of research published through January 2009. *Osteoarthritis Cartilage*. 2010;18:476-499.

22   Baker KR, Nelson ME, Felson DT, Layne JE, Sarno R, Roubenoff R. The efficacy of home based progressive strength training in older adults with knee osteoarthritis: a randomized controlled trial. *J Rheumatol*. 2001;28:1655-1665.

23   Ettinger WH Jr, Burns R, Messier SP, et al. A randomized trial comparing aerobic exercise and resistance exercise with a health education program in older adults with knee osteoarthritis. The Fitness Arthritis and Seniors Trial (FAST). *JAMA*. 1997;277:25-31.

24   O'Reilly SC, Muir KR, Doherty M. Effectiveness of home exercise on pain and disability from osteoarthritis of the knee: a randomised controlled trial. *Ann Rheum Dis*. 1999;58:15-19.

25   Røgind H, Bibow-Nielsen B, Jensen B, Møller HC, Frimodt-Møller H, Bliddal H. The effects of a physical training program on patients with osteoarthritis of the knees. *Arch Phys Med Rehabil*. 1998;79:1421-1427.

26   Fisher NM, Gresham GE, Abrams M, Hicks J, Horrigan D, Pendergast DR. Quantitative effects of physical therapy on muscular and functional performance in subjects with osteoarthritis of the knees. *Arch Phys Med Rehabil*. 1993;74:840-847.

27   Baker K, McAlindon T. Exercise for knee osteoarthritis. *Curr Opin Rheumatol*. 2000;12:456-463.

28 Fisher NM, White SC, Yack HJ, Smolinski RJ, Pendergast DR. Muscle function and gait in patients with knee osteoarthritis before and after muscle rehabilitation. *Disabil Rehabil.* 1997;19:47-55.

29 Bennell KL, Hunt MA, Wrigley TV, Lim BW, Hinman RS. Role of muscle in the genesis and management of knee osteoarthritis. *Rheum Dis Clin North Am.* 2008;34:731-754.

30 Bennell KL, Hunter DJ, Hinman RS. Management of osteoarthritis of the knee. *BMJ.* 2012;345:e4934.

31 Gross KD, Hillstrom HJ. Noninvasive devices targeting the mechanics of osteoarthritis. *Rheum Dis Clin North Am.* 2008;34:755-776.

32 Gross KD. Device use: walking aids, braces, and orthoses for symptomatic knee osteoarthritis. *Clin Geriatr Med.* 2010;26:479-502.

33 Harvey WF, Hunter DJ. The role of analgesics and intra-articular injections in disease management. *Rheum Dis Clin North Am.* 2008;34:777-788.

34 Lo GH, LaValley M, McAlindon T, Felson DT. Intra-articular hyaluronic acid in treatment of knee osteoarthritis: a meta-analysis. *JAMA.* 2003;290:3115-3121.

35 Clegg DO, Reda DJ, Harris CL, et al. Glucosamine, chondroitin sulfate, and the two in combination for painful knee osteoarthritis. *N Engl J Med.* 2006;354:795-808.

36 Ortiz E. Market withdrawal of Vioxx: is it time to rethink the use of COX-2 inhibitors? *J Manag Care Pharm.* 2004;10:551-554.

37 Bookman AA, Williams KS, Shainhouse JZ. Effect of a topical diclofenac solution for relieving symptoms of primary osteoarthritis of the knee: a randomized controlled trial. *CMAJ.* 2004;171:333-338.

38 Lin J, Zhang W, Jones A, Doherty M. Efficacy of topical non-steroidal anti-inflammatory drugs in the treatment of osteoarthritis: meta-analysis of randomised controlled trials. *BMJ.* 2004;329:324.

39 Altman R, Barkin RL. Topical therapy for osteoarthritis: clinical and pharmacologic perspectives. *Postgrad Med.* 2009;121:139-147.

40 Conaghan P, Birrell F, Burke M, et al; Guideline Development Group for The National Collaborating Centre for Chronic Conditions. *Osteoarthritis: National Clinical Guideline for Care and Management in Adults.* London, UK: Royal College of Physicians; 2008.

41 Harvey WF, Hunter DJ. Pharmacologic intervention for osteoarthritis in older adults. *Clin Geriatr Med.* 2010;26:503-515.

42 Case JP, Baliunas AJ, Block JA. Lack of efficacy of acetaminophen in treating symptomatic knee osteoarthritis: a randomized, double-blind, placebo-controlled comparison trial with diclofenac sodium. *Arch Intern Med.* 2003;163:169-178.

43 Golden HE, Moskowitz RW, Minic M. Analgesic efficacy and safety of nonprescription doses of naproxen sodium compared with acetaminophen in the treatment of osteoarthritis of the knee. *Am J Ther.* 2004;11:85-94.

44 Miceli-Richard C, Le Bars M, Schmidely N, Dougados M. Paracetamol in osteoarthritis of the knee. *Ann Rheum Dis.* 2004;63:923-930.

45 Pincus T, Koch G, Lei H, et al. Patient Preference for Placebo, Acetaminophen (paracetamol) or Celecoxib Efficacy Studies (PACES): two randomised, double blind, placebo controlled, crossover clinical trials in patients with knee or hip osteoarthritis. *Ann Rheum Dis.* 2004;63:931-939.

46 Pincus T, Swearingen C, Cummins P, Callahan LF. Preference for nonsteroidal antiinflammatory drugs versus acetaminophen and concomitant use of both types of drugs in patients with osteoarthritis. *J Rheumatol.* 2000;27:1020-1027.

47 Herrero-Beaumont G, Ivorra JA, Del Carmen Trabado M, et al. Glucosamine sulfate in the treatment of knee osteoarthritis symptoms: a randomized, double-blind, placebo-controlled study using acetaminophen as a side comparator. *Arthritis Rheum.* 2007;56:555-567.

48 Massó González EL, Patrignani P, Tacconelli S, García Rodríguez LA. Variability among nonsteroidal antiinflammatory drugs in risk of upper gastrointestinal bleeding. *Arthritis Rheum.* 2010;62:1592-1601.

49 McGettigan P, Henry D. Cardiovascular risk and inhibition of cyclooxygenase: a systematic review of the observational studies of selective and nonselective inhibitors of cyclooxygenase 2. *JAMA.* 2006;296:1633-1644.

50 Rao PNP, Knaus EE. Evolution of nonsteroidal anti-inflammatory drugs (NSAIDs): cyclooxygenase (COX) inhibition and beyond. *J Pharm Pharm Sci.* 2008;11:81s-110s.

51 Patrignani P, Tacconelli S, Bruno A, Sostres C, Lanas A. Managing the adverse effects of nonsteroidal anti-inflammatory drugs. *Expert Rev Clin Pharmacol.* 2011;4:605-621.

52 Lanas A, Garcia-Rodriguez LA, Polo-Tomás M, et al. Time trends and impact of upper and lower gastrointestinal bleeding and perforation in clinical practice. *Am J Gastroenterol.* 2009;104:1633-1641.

53 Trelle S, Reichenbach S, Wandel S, et al. Cardiovascular safety of non-steroidal anti-inflammatory drugs: network meta-analysis. *BMJ.* 2011;342:c7086.

54 Bellamy N, Campbell J, Robinson V, Gee T, Bourne R, Wells G. Intraarticular corticosteroid for treatment of osteoarthritis of the knee. *Cochrane Database Syst Rev.* 2005;CD005328.

55 Rutjes AW, Jüni P, da Costa BR, Trelle S, Nüesch E, Reichenbach S. Viscosupplementation for osteoarthritis of the knee: a systematic review and meta-analysis. *Ann Intern Med.* 2012;157:180-191.

56 Chappell AS, Desaiah D, Liu-Seifert H, et al. A double-blind, randomized, placebo-controlled study of the efficacy and safety of duloxetine for the treatment of chronic pain due to osteoarthritis of the knee. *Pain Pract.* 2011;11:33-41.

57 Bijlsma JWJ, Berenbaum F, Lafeber FPJG. Osteoarthritis: an update with relevance for clinical practice. *Lancet.* 2011;377:2115-2126.

58 Hochberg MC. Structure-modifying effects of chondroitin sulfate in knee osteoarthritis: an updated meta-analysis of randomized placebo-controlled trials of 2-year duration. *Osteoarthritis Cartilage.* 2010;18:S28-S31.

59 Matthews GL, Hunter DJ. Emerging drugs for osteoarthritis. *Expert Opin Emerg Drugs.* 2011;16:479-491.

60 Hunter DJ. Pharmacologic therapy for osteoarthritis – the era of disease modification. *Nat Rev Rheumatol.* 2011;7:13-22.

61 Richmond JC. Surgery for osteoarthritis of the knee. *Rheum Dis Clin North Am.* 2008;34:815-825.

62 Hall MJ, Lawrence L. Ambulatory surgery in the United States, 1996. *Adv Data.* 1998;300:1-16.

63 Brinker MR, O'Connor DP, Pierce P, Woods GW, Elliott MN. Utilization of orthopaedic services in a capitated population. *J Bone Joint Surg Am.* 2002;84-A:1926-1932.

64 Moseley JB, O'Malley K, Petersen NJ, et al. A controlled trial of arthroscopic surgery for osteoarthritis of the knee. *N Engl J Med.* 2002;347:81-88.

65 Kirkley A, Birmingham TB, Litchfield RB, et al. A randomized trial of arthroscopic surgery for osteoarthritis of the knee. *N Engl J Med.* 2008;359:1097-1107.

66 Brouwer RW, Bierma-Zeinstra SMA, Verhagen AP, Jakma TSC, Verhaar JAN. Osteotomy for treating knee osteoarthritis. *Cochrane Database Syst Rev.* 2007;(3):CD004019.

67 Naudie D, Bourne RB, Rorabeck CH, Bourne TJ. The Insall Award. Survivorship of the high tibial valgus osteotomy. A 10- to -22-year follow-up study. *Clin Orthop Relat Res.* 1999;367:18-27.

68 Stukenborg-Colsman C, Wirth CJ, Lazovic D, Wefer A. High tibial osteotomy versus unicompartmental joint replacement in unicompartmental knee joint osteoarthritis: 7–10-year follow-up prospective randomised study. *Knee.* 2001;8:187-194.

69 Mancuso CA, Ranawat CS, Esdaile JM, Johanson NA, Charlson ME. Indications for total hip and total knee arthroplasties. Results of orthopaedic surveys. *J Arthroplasty.* 1996;11:34-46.

70 Fortin PR, Clarke AE, Joseph L, et al. Outcomes of total hip and knee replacement: preoperative functional status predicts outcomes at six months after surgery. *Arthritis Rheum.* 1999;42:1722-1728.

Printed by Printforce, the Netherlands